FEELING
Good . . .

by Sara Gilbert

Feeling Good . . .

A Book About You and Your Body

Four Winds Press New York

LIBRARY OF CONGRESS CATALOGING IN PUBLICATION DATA

Gilbert, Sara D
    Feeling good: a book about you and your body.

    Bibliography: p.
    SUMMARY: Discusses physical, emotional, and mental changes that occur during adolescence and how to care for one's body and cope with problems and conditions that might occur.
    1. Adolescence—Juvenile literature. 2. Youth—Health and hygiene—Juvenile literature. [1. Adolescence. 2. Health] I. Title.
RJ140.G54   613'.04'33   78–5306
ISBN 0–590–07510–1

Published by Four Winds Press
A division of Scholastic Magazines, Inc., New York, N.Y.
Copyright © 1978 by Sara Gilbert
All rights reserved
Printed in the United States of America
Library of Congress Catalog Card Number: 78–5306
1 2 3 4 5 82 81 80 79 78

This book is for Sean, tomorrow.

CONTENTS

aCKNOWLEdGMENTS

Very special thanks are owed to S. Kenneth Schonberg, M.D., Assistant Director of the Division of Adolescent Medicine at Montefiore Hospital (New York City), for his careful reading of the manuscript and for his valuable suggestions and contributions.

The author is also grateful to Dr. Barry Goldberg of the Institute of Sports Medicine and Athletic Trauma at Lenox Hill Hospital (New York City); to Dr. Adele Hoffman, adolescent specialist at the New York University Medical Center; to Dr. Ralph Lopez of New York Hospital's adolescent division; and to Dr. Lucie Rudd, chief of adolescent medicine at Roosevelt Hospital (New York City), for their time, information, and ideas.

1

THE NEW YOU

This book is about your body—how it works, why it's changing, how to cope with some of the problems it is likely to give you, and how you can learn to work with your body rather than against it so that you can keep feeling good.

Your body is undergoing a major transformation: it is turning you from a child into an adult. (Adolescence literally means "becoming adult.") New hormones—the chemicals that regulate the body's activities—are flowing through your bloodstream, and as a result you look different on the outside and you function, feel, and perhaps even think differently on the inside from the way you did when you were younger.

At this stage in your life, when you are about to enter adolescence, you probably find that you have a lot more questions about your body than you ever had had before. When you were a little kid, you may not have been really aware of your body. Perhaps you learned about the parts and systems of the human body in grade school, but your own body was probably of less interest. Most children simply use their bodies without thinking about them. But now, you may find that you are thinking about your body a lot, and it is changing so fast and in such surprising ways that it's hard to ignore.

Did you know that between the ages of ten and sixteen, girls on the average gain fifty pounds and grow nine inches? Boys add an average of sixty pounds and ten inches from age twelve to age eighteen. That is more growing than you have done since you were an infant.

Often, this growth comes in sudden spurts: in a single year you may grow through several sizes of clothes. And it's not only your size that's changing, but your surface as well—boys get harder and girls get softer. Your body may be changing shape, too, and sprouting hair in odd places. Your face looks different. You smell different. You feel different. So it is no wonder that many people your age feel like strangers in their own bodies.

As your body is growing up, so are you. Until now, it has been your parents' job to see that you ate well, got enough sleep, played enough in the "fresh air" and received proper medical care. Your family is still concerned about your health and physical well-being, of course, but they no longer have the kind of control over you and your body that they once did.

As you become more independent, you will begin to feed yourself whatever you want and refuse to eat whatever meals you don't care for. You can go to sleep whenever you're ready. You can spend your free time doing whatever you want to. Your parents may not be happy that they can no longer force you to do what they think is best for you. But like it or not, that's the way it is.

More and more, what you do *to* and *for* your body is up to you. The more facts and the fewer myths you can apply, the better off you and your body will be. For instance, did you know a lot of the old rules for good health have changed? Some of the kinds of exercise that we've always assumed were good for us may actually be dangerous. Getting a proper diet can be trickier in these days of fortified wonder foods and chemical creations than it was when all we had to think about was three square meals from four food groups. You may be surprised to learn that good nutrition does not mean three square meals a day.

The concept of "clean living" has taken on new definitions now that the straight and narrow path seems to have added a lot of detours. If we can't go by the old rules, each of us may need to find our own "rules" for feeling good. This book will serve as an introductory guide to help you decide how to take care of yourself.

This book is also about your "self." Your body is, of course, a major part of "you." For one thing, you would simply not exist without your body. If it is sick, you can't function. The better it works, the better off you are.

But your self is wrapped up in your body in other, less obvious ways. Although it is sometimes hard to make the connection between our mental and emotional life and our physical state, our thoughts and feelings *are* connected to the organs, cells, and fluids of our bodies. They have to be, for they are all part of the same package. You can *feel good*—feel good about yourself, feel good about your body, and just plain feel good—by finding out all you can about your body, your mind, and your emotions and by learning how to make them all work together for *you*.

Most of us tend to be very private about our bodies. We are taught to cover them with clothing, and so we are often embarrassed to discuss or even to think about those hidden but all-important parts of our selves. Most of us at one time or another have some aspect of our bodies that causes us shame or concern but that we feel is too private to talk or ask about.

This book contains information about many problems that often especially trouble people your age. If you have a particular worry or a specific question, you can find out more about it, privately, by looking up that topic in the table of contents or the index. You may be surprised and perhaps relieved to realize that "your" problem is one that many people share.

2

"why am i so ugly?"

Do you spend more time looking in the mirror than you used to? Probably—most people your age do. And do you like everything you see? Probably not—most teen-agers find something in their appearance to hate. Early adolescence is not a time when people's bodies look their best. There are a number of physical characteristics considered "irregular" according to some ideal standard of beauty that are common to most people at your stage of life.

❧ Gangliness. Do you look like an ostrich, with a long scrawny neck and gangly, awkward-looking limbs? There's no point in running to hide your head in the sand. The fact is that during adolescence the neck, arms and legs do grow faster than the rest of the body. This growth pattern is one reason why you may become unusually clumsy, bumping into things and tripping over your feet.

❧   Pudginess. Are you a "fat blob"? You may never have been fat before in your life, and all of a sudden you seem like one big pudge. Chances are you're being overcritical, but you may actually be temporarily fatter than you once were. Early adolescence is a time when many people add a layer of "puppy fat." Girls may notice it particularly in their abdomens; boys may be especially aware of fat in their upper thighs or around their nipples. Or the body may just look soft all over. Exactly why some early teens look like butterballs is not known for certain; it might be the result of hormone changes in the body.

❧   Scrawniness. Or do you see a "scrawny skeleton" in your mirror? Perhaps you've always been thin and are only just noticing it now. But your skinny look may be a new thing, and it, too, can be quite normal. You may be gaining height so rapidly now that your body lacks the reserves to keep itself padded. That will change when your growth slows. In fact, for a few years some young people alternate being skinny and fat.

❧   Changing skin. Do you have "hideous skin"? Many teen-agers have acne; but even if your skin is clear, it may seem coarse and greasy. It's not your imagination. Your pores *are* larger than they once were, and your skin *is* producing more oil. That too is the result of hormone shifts in your body.

❧   New hair. It is hard to imagine anyone of any age who is completely satisfied with the texture, color, or thickness of his or her hair. Not only that, but your hair is probably different from what it once was. The cute little golden curls you had when you were younger may have turned mousey and straight; or the straight brown stuff you remember from childhood may have been replaced by a kinky tangled mess. Not everyone's hair changes are so dramatic, but hair does tend to become darker, coarser, and thicker—and oilier, too—in adolescence. The newness may be startling, and you may be discouraged if your type of hair won't bend to the style you're dying for.

Of course, it isn't the hair on your head that makes the strangest changes in your mirror image. The fine film of hairs around your genitals may have been the first sign that you were no longer a little kid. "Puberty," a word that overlaps in many ways with "adolescence," comes from the Latin word *pubes* (pronounced "pew-beze"), meaning the hair that grows in the groin or crotch. The hair on your arms and legs is probably also becoming denser and more noticeable, and this too is a sign that you will soon be an adult.

Many girls may be alarmed to see hair sprouting around their nipples, in a line up toward their belly-button, or in a shadow over their upper lip. This does not mean that there is something wrong with you. All humans have some elements of both "maleness" and "femaleness" in them, and as your adult hormones go into action the "male" ones give you hair where only boys are "supposed" to have it.

Boys in their early teens may panic that they will never grow a beard or get hair on their chests; but chest and facial hair tend to appear late in adolescent development, so relax. In the meantime, take your eye off the mirror and think about the men in your family. Is your father, grandfather, uncle, or older brother hairy or not? That will give you some idea of what hair you can expect when the time is right. Most Black, Oriental, and Indian men have little or no chest hair, and many Caucasian families tend to be hairless. Body hair has nothing to do with "manliness."

❧   Strange smells. You can't see your odors, but you probably can smell a lot of new ones on your body. Your perspiration didn't used to smell; now it does. You tend to notice that odor mostly in your armpits, but actually your entire body smells different from the way it did when you were younger. Your urine has a strong odor, too: this is especially noticeable among boys, but girls experience it as well. And a girl's vaginal secretions also may have an odor for the first time.

A DIFFERENT SHAPE

As you grow through adolescence, your skeleton will probably change shape dramatically. Boys develop broader chests and shoulders; girls widen through the hips. Even your face may look different as the bones shift from a structure "designed" to meet an infant's needs to one better suited to an adult's intake of food and air.

You may be dissatisfied with the new you in the mirror because it's not in the shape it's "supposed" to be. The adult bodies you've seen all your life in movies and magazines and on television all curve and bulge in the "right" places. And now that you are getting an adult body, maybe it doesn't look the way those ideal shapes do. Well, there's no need for panic—there's nothing wrong with you. Few adults have "ideal" shapes, and those who do get paid a lot of money to show them off and keep them up. For a better idea of what shape is "normal" for you, take a close look at the men and women in your family; that will show you what kind of body you can expect to grow into.

New smells, new shapes, new texture, new hair— you've got a lot of newness to become familiar with. But while you're looking at your changing reflection, remember another characteristic that many teen-agers share: they are overly critical of themselves. It is as though, now that they are for the first time really aware of themselves as individuals, they want those individuals to be absolutely perfect.

It's natural to want to look your best; just don't tear yourself down when you find a "flaw." If you are worried about your hair, for instance, you may concentrate on it until it seems to be worse than it really is, just as when you stare at a word long enough or write it over and over again, it seems to be misspelled. Although you may firmly believe that no one else in the world could possibly have such ugly hair, your particular "flaw" is probably something that millions of people your age are also worried about.

UGLY IS AS UGLY FEELS

Take another look at that reflection in the mirror. What you see there can affect how you feel about yourself. That makes sense, doesn't it? If you think that your body is generally attractive, that helps you to feel okay about yourself; if you think that your body looks ugly or silly, you may not feel so good.

And it works the other way, too. Let's imagine Alf and Harry. They're both small for their age, both are a little underweight, and each has a long, thin neck that makes his large head seem even bigger than it is. Let's say that Alf likes himself: he's pretty happy, usually successful at what he tries, and his family and friends think he's an all-right guy. The body he sees in his mirror he calls "slender" and "compact." And his big head only shows how "brainy" he is.

Harry, on the other hand, is going through a time when he feels rotten about himself. He's doing poorly in school, and didn't make the track team. His best friend just moved away, and his father's always on his back about something. So when he looks at himself in the mirror, the body he sees is "puny" and "scrawny," and his head and neck make him look like a "freak."

Alf has what's called a "positive body image," and Harry has a "negative body image." That is another way of saying that the way we feel about ourselves influences the way we look to ourselves, and the way we think we look has a lot to do with the way we behave—since Alf thinks he looks like a winner, he is more apt to act like, and perhaps be, a winner.

YOU ARE HOW YOU LOOK

We are taught that we shouldn't "judge a book by its cover"; that "clothes don't make the man," and that "beauty is only skin deep." We are taught all that, but we still tend to evaluate people's personalities and characters by their appearance, and we in turn are judged by how we look. In a way, this isn't fair. It certainly wouldn't be fair, for instance, to decide that a girl was worthless just because her hair was straggly, or that a boy was stupid because he had acne. But in another way, it can be said that you are how you look. Your appearance often can express what kind of person you are and how you are feeling.

A smiling face, of course, indicates a happy mood; a frowning face signals gloom or anger. When you see a guy slumping along, with hanging head and dragging feet, you would say that he is "down." His whole body is expressing the weight of his depression. And a gal with her head and shoulders held high and with a lift to her walk is showing through her body that she is in an "up" mood.

But appearance can offer clues to more than different moods. Spend some time just watching people on the street and see how much you can tell about their personalities from how they look. A man who walks, shoulders back and head high, with a firm, brisk gait, comes across as strong, proud, and purposeful. A man who stoops, hangs his head, and shuffles seems timid, weak, and unsure of himself. A woman whose face is haggard, whose hair is a mess, and whose clothes are sloppy may be telling the world that she is ashamed of her body and of herself. The perfect hairdo and makeup and the beautifully fitting clothes on another woman may be signs that she wants people to notice her.

Such judgments of passersby may be completely wrong, of course. The first man may be trying hard to "keep his chin up" because he feels rotten; the second woman may be so unhappy with who she is that she needs to put on a "mask" of makeup and a "costume" of fancy clothing to conceal her true feelings. But in *some* way, the way people care for and present their bodies is usually a sign of who they are and how they feel about themselves.

WHAT TYPE ARE YOU?

There's even a psychological theory that relates personality to body type. This "somatotype" system (*soma* is the Greek word for body) classifies people as endomorphs, mesomorphs, and ectomorphs. Endomorphs appear fat rather than bony or muscular; mesomorphs are stocky and well muscled; ectomorphs are thin and bony looking. According to the somatotype theory of personality, endomorphs are sociable, easygoing, and pleasure-loving; mesomorphs are aggressive, athletic, and energetic; and ectomorphs are "brainy," nervous, and shy.

Classifying personalities by body type has caused a lot of argument. It would be pretty discouraging, after all, to think that because of the shapes of our bodies we were forever stuck with the personalities that were "supposed" to go with them.

Yet even people who've never heard of the somatotype theory have probably used the system themselves. When we meet a chubby woman for the first time, we may tend to assume that she is jolly and fun-loving, and we behave toward her as though she is. After a while, she learns, perhaps without realizing it, that acting jolly and fun-loving is the best way to deal with the people she meets. When we meet a skinny, weak-looking man, we often react by keeping our distance, and that kind of treatment would make anybody shy and nervous.

At the very least the theory is a way of saying that the way we feel and live shows itself in our bodies. An energetic, busy person would tend to develop more muscles than a lazier one. An easygoing, self-indulgent person would indeed tend to be pudgy. Someone who is nervous and withdrawn would probably not develop the fat and the muscles to change that bony look. Whatever you think of the somatotype theory, you probably agree that our outside appearance and our inside selves do interact.

3

TOO SHORT, TOO TALL, TOO SOMETHING

On her way to Wonderland, Alice drank from a magic bottle and became very small. Then she ate a magic cake and grew very tall. Many people your age must feel like Alice—they feel either too short or too tall. But there's no magic potion to blame; your growth rate and patterns are built right into your system and have been since long before you were born.

Overall human growth and development, however, generally follow a definite sequence. Typical development progresses in stages, no matter at what age it occurs. That is, no matter how old she is, a girl probably can't expect to menstruate until her breasts start to develop; a boy of any age needn't look for chest hair until he has a crop of pubic hair. The charts on page 18 show the different stages of adolescent growth and development. Notice that the body's fastest gain in height begins shortly after the first appearance of pubic hair. That means that while you are "growing up," you are also *growing*.

THE GROWTH GLANDS

Exactly what triggers this growth spurt, or what keeps it from happening sooner, is not thoroughly understood, but scientists have gained a fairly clear picture of the process.

During childhood, an uncharted intersection in the front part of your brain works with the hypothalamus and the pineal, two tiny sections of the center of your brain, to prevent your body from maturing.

Then at some point the growth inhibitors let go of the reins. The hypothalamus stimulates the body's "master gland," the pituitary, to send growth signals to the thyroid and adrenal glands, the gonads, and other glands that regulate development. The end result of the chain reaction is that you start growing.

Although most people grow at their maximum rate just before their reproductive organs begin to function, they don't do all their growing at once. You may notice that you seem to stop growing for a while and then all of a sudden get too tall for your clothes again. These growth spurts occur because once the gonads (the reproductive glands: ovaries in females and testes in males) get into gear, their hormones signal the other glands to stop sending "grow!" messages. But when the level of sex hormones falls below a certain level, the pituitary gets busy again, and you grow a bit more. Eventually the system balances out, development stops, and the "growth glands" function only to maintain the body of stimulating the replacement of worn-out cells, rather than to increase its size.

Usually all parts of the body don't grow at the same time. Your neck, arms, and legs will probably gain length first, while at a different time you may grow through your torso so that your ribs are lifted off your pelvis and your body is longer from the hips to the shoulders than it was when you were younger.

You're not only gaining height during these growth spurts. Your bones are growing and becoming heavier as soft cartilage turns into solid material. Your shoulders and rib cage are expanding to make room for larger adult organs, and in girls the pelvic bone is widening. To be able to move these heavier bones, your muscles are also growing in size. So by the time your growth has stopped, you are not only taller than you were a few years before, but you are broader and heavier, too.

WHEN WILL I EVER START GROWING?

But when can you expect all this growth to occur? The growing and changing can, in themselves, be troublesome enough, and the timing of it all only adds to the difficulty.

As the charts on page 18 show, the biggest growth spurt begins about a year after the onset of puberty has been signaled by the first growth of pubic hair. But that's hardly an answer because puberty begins at a different time for each individual. The onset of puberty and the growth spurt are, the experts assume, programmed into you by the genes you inherited from your parents.

One pattern that is typical is that girls mature earlier than boys, beginning at ages ranging from nine to twelve, with an average age of eleven to thirteen. Of course, a given individual might be older than twelve or younger than nine at the start of her physical adolescence, so that she might start her growth spurt as young as eight and still be considered "normal." Boys on the average begin to mature sometime from eleven to sixteen, most often at about twelve, so they don't start their extra-rapid growth until about age eleven.

Beginning in about the fourth or fifth grade, you probably noticed that girls are taller than boys. That's because of the different maturation rates. You were probably unaware of it when you were younger, but from birth on (and according to some theories, even before birth) the girls you know have been maturing faster than the boys. Little girls, for instance, have better control over their small muscles (such as those in their fingers) sooner than little boys do. But girls stop growing at a younger age, too, so boys catch up in height and other signs of maturation later in adolescence.

Knowing that you are going to catch up in a few years doesn't help if you're in love with the girl who sits next to you, and you feel like a kid because she's two feet taller than you are. Or no matter how good a

GIRL'S ADOLESCENT DEVELOPMENT SEQUENCE
earliest beginning: age 8

	begins	+6 months	+1 year	+1½ years	+2 years	+2½ years	+3 years	ends
Pubic Hair	≈≈	≈≈	≈≈	≈≈	≈≈	≈≈	≈≈	≈≈
Breast Growth	≈≈	≈≈	≈≈	≈≈	≈≈	≈≈	≈≈	≈≈
Height Spurt				≈≈	≈≈	≈≈	≈≈	≈≈
1st Menstruation					≈≈	≈≈		
Pelvic Growth/ "Hips"					≈≈	≈≈	≈≈	≈≈
1st Ovulation*							≈≈	≈≈

BOY'S ADOLESCENT DEVELOPMENT SEQUENCE
earliest beginning: age 10

	begins	+6 months	+1 year	+1½ years	+2 years	+2½ years	+3 years	+3½ years	+4 years	ends
Pubic Hair	≈≈	≈≈	≈≈	≈≈	≈≈	≈≈	≈≈	≈≈	≈≈	≈≈
Testes Growth	≈≈	≈≈	≈≈	≈≈	≈≈	≈≈	≈≈	≈≈	≈≈	≈≈
Height Spurt			≈≈	≈≈	≈≈	≈≈	≈≈	≈≈	≈≈	≈≈
Penis Growth			≈≈	≈≈	≈≈	≈≈	≈≈	≈≈	≈≈	≈≈
Voice Change					≈≈	≈≈	≈≈	≈≈	≈≈	≈≈
Semen Production*						≈≈	≈≈	≈≈	≈≈	≈≈
Face and Body Hair					≈≈	≈≈	≈≈	≈≈	≈≈	≈≈

* Watch out! These are *average* timings for the production of the first egg and sperm cells. You cannot assume that there is a "safe" time after your first menstruation or your first ejaculation.

dancer you are, you're definitely going to feel clumsy dancing with some guy you can hardly see. There's nothing you can do about such awkward situations except to be patient or to decide that a person's height doesn't make much difference.

But not every girl grows sooner than every boy; the pattern varies from person to person. Within each sex, too, maturation timing varies widely. You and your best friend may once have been taken for twins, until she, apparently overnight, got twice as tall as you. Or you may grow almost tall enough to touch the basketball net, while the guy your age next door is still about the right height for playing marbles. If your friends are growing and you're not, or if you're towering over all your classmates, it doesn't mean that there's something wrong with you. It's just that everyone is different. You can get a good idea of when you'll grow or stop growing and how tall you'll eventually be by asking your parents about their growth as teen-agers. If your father was an early maturer, or your mother a late bloomer during his or her adolescence, the chances are that you will follow their patterns. If you are still concerned about not growing or about growing too much, ask your doctor. A doctor familiar with adolescent development can measure your height, weight, and bone size against your particular stage of sexual development and be able to give you a pretty good prediction of when you'll achieve your eventual size.

4

"do i HAVE TO GROW UP?"

You may think, I was happy as a kid. No one asked me to wash the dishes; no one worried about my getting a job, or getting into college. Why do I have to grow up? The answer is simple: you're growing so that you will be big enough to produce and care for offspring. We are, after all, basically animals and our bodies are governed by the laws of nature. As far as Mother Nature is concerned, the only purpose of human life is the reproduction of more human life.

Remember that growth is caused in part by the reproductive glands. Physical growth and sexual maturation go together; the same hormones that stimulate your bones to grow also stir your reproductive system into operation. While you are watching the outside of your body grow, the inside is changing, too. Shortly after their growth slows most teen-agers are capable of reproducing.

A girl is said to be sexually mature when she begins to ovulate, when her ovaries first release an egg cell or ovum. A boy is mature sexually as soon as his body begins to produce sperm cells (he is capable of ejaculating fluid from his penis before that, but the ejaculate contains no sperm). At that point, from the standpoint of biology, a boy and a girl can become parents; and if we were cave people, they probably would be parents at an early age. So their bodies must be big enough and strong enough to give birth, to carry and protect their young, and to kill food for their families.

SIGNS OF CHANGE

The outward signs of these internal changes are called "secondary sex characteristics." Primary sex characteristics are the internal changes themselves, the functioning ovaries and testes. The secondary characteristics are visible evidence of this activity.

Some of these signs are the same for both boys and girls. Both boys and girls develop hair around the genitals and under the arms. First it is thin and soft, but it gradually becomes coarse and thick. The hair already growing on the rest of the body becomes denser, too. (Why should specialized body hair be a key sign of adulthood? Nobody knows for sure, but it seems reasonable to assume that it is a remaining trace of our basic animal nature. The plumage and coats of birds and beasts change as they mature, and become signals to other members of the species that an individual creature is old enough to mate.)

Also, the voices of both boys and girls drop into a lower register, though this change is more obvious in boys. The genitals of both sexes grow in size, although boys will usually notice this change in their bodies more than girls will.

There are, of course, differences in secondary sex characteristics. Girls enter adolescence about two years earlier than boys. A girl's first sign that she is changing as well as growing is that her breasts begin to develop, starting with the nipples, which become darker and pointier. During development, the breasts are often sensitive or painful, but the discomfort disappears with maturity.

The most dramatic symptom of a girl's adolescence is her first period, or menstruation. This is a sign that the uterus, or womb, is capable of receiving a fertilized egg cell and nurturing it through pregnancy. Menstruation is a word derived from the Latin word for month, because it occurs approximately once a month in female adults. (Don't be alarmed if you don't menstruate every month at first. It takes time for most girls to establish a regular monthly cycle.)

The bloody discharge of menstruation is the special layer of cells that develops on the walls of the uterus each month in preparation for the fetus or developing baby that would attach there if an egg were released and fertilized. When a fertilized egg is not attached, the lining is not needed, and the body discards it.

The other changes in a girl's body are less dramatic, but more noticeable to the world at large. Her pelvic bones widen and shift position, making it possible to give birth to a baby and giving her "hips" for the first time. And she adds a soft layer of body fat which will stay with her. Women's bodies tend to have more fat than men's, perhaps because nature intended them to be comfortable for their babies.

A boy may first realize that he is on the way to manhood when his testes "drop." In normal development, the sperm-producing organs called testes or balls actually descend into the scrotum, the sac that holds them, just before birth. But at puberty, both the testes and the scrotum grow so rapidly that they seem to have "dropped." The testes are located outside of the body because sperm cannot develop at the body's normal internal temperature, and the scrotum expands and contracts according to the external temperature to keep the testes at a more or less constant warmth. The penis grows rapidly as well, and becomes capable of ejaculating, or squirting out, fluid secreted by the prostate gland and other parts of the reproductive tract. When this fluid contains sperm cells, it is called semen.

A boy's chest and shoulders broaden during puberty, and his body becomes more muscular. He gradually develops facial hair, and at about the time the internal shifts are complete, he may begin to sprout chest hair. It is because chest hair, if it appears at all, is the last secondary sex characteristic to develop that some people mistakenly consider it a sign of virility or "manliness."

"AM I GROWING RIGHT?"

The development of such characteristics of biological maturity as breasts or body hair is often the source of a great deal of concern for teen-agers.

Part of the problem is that growth and development happen at different ages for different people. Girls get embarrassed about developing breasts sooner than their friends, or worry if they are still flat-chested when their friends are busty. Boys may panic if they aren't becoming "men" as soon as their classmates, or may feel intensely uncomfortable at having to associate with girls who are, for a time, much older looking than they are. Remember that each body develops according to its own genetically programmed pattern and speed. Everyone matures eventually; some people just start earlier than others.

If Mary has started to menstruate and you haven't, or if John is shaving and you're still in peach fuzz, there's nothing wrong with you. But that kind of thing can be a worry. So many strange and remarkable things are happening to your body that it is perfectly natural for a person your age to wonder if what's happening is normal, if you are "growing right." The charts on page 18 outlining the sequence of physical maturation should give you a general idea of the course your body is following and of the changes you can expect.

CHILD OR ADULT?

But physical maturation doesn't always parallel social maturation, and this situation can cause extra problems. Although your body may be physically ready for parenthood and adult sexual activity, your parents and the society they represent still consider you a child.

Adults try to restrict you because they know or feel that, whether you're biologically mature or not, you still have a lot more growing up to do by society's standards. Your parents are telling you one thing, and your body is "telling" you another.

5

"AM i A SEX MANiAC?"

A lot of what your body is telling you probably has to do with sex. Sex is a source of worry for practically every teen-ager—whether it's too much, not enough, the "wrong kind," or just confusion about the facts.

This chapter assumes that you have a basic understanding of the facts of the reproductive process; that you know where babies come from and how they are made. Just to make sure, though, you might want to check out some of the books listed on pages 157–160.

Many people your age complain that neither their schools nor their parents provide enough sex education; and even if you think you know it all, you might learn some new facts. Surprisingly few adults, no matter how great their experience, have a complete understanding of the reproductive process.

BEHIND THE DRIVE

For many young people, sexual feelings and urges are in themselves a cause for concern. The sensations may be new and unfamiliar, although it is quite common and natural for young children to have sexual urges. They are certainly new in their intensity, and this can be bewildering. A boy may find that he gets an erection at the slightest erotic thought or suggestion. A girl may feel a response in her genitals to situations that suggest sex or romance.

These reactions can often cause confusion, embarrassment, or even shame. They needn't. All humans have a drive, an inborn push, to reproduce; *nature's* only purpose for our lives is the reproduction of our own kind. Sexual intercourse is the means by which we achieve that purpose. Your body is ready for reproduction, or almost so. So it is natural that you feel the sensations that signal the force of the reproductive drive.

LOVE TALK

Sexual stirrings are often accompanied by feelings of love. Like sex urges, romantic love—love for a person other than a family member—usually also first appears in a person's life during early adolescence.

Falling in love is an important activity of adolescence, the experts say, because it gives young people "practice" for the mature love relationships they will enter as adults, and because forming close attachments is a way of easing the separation from parental control. Having a close relationship with another person is also a good way of learning about one's self, and the formation of an identity is another vital psychological task of adolescence.

These explanations may make sense, but no one can really explain love, or take away its magic by giving it a reason. Falling in love is one of the most pleasant and sometimes one of the most painful of all human experiences. When it happens, nothing else seems to matter. And that makes the conflicts between the body's urges and society's rules all the harder to resolve.

RIGHT AND WRONG

As humans, we are not governed by nature alone. Nor does the world revolve around love. Falling in love may be nature's way of encouraging us to reproduce, but our society and culture provide rules and standards that have at least as much power over our behavior as nature's "laws."

In general, society does not approve of sexual activity that takes place outside a legal marriage. A major purpose of this rule has been to insure that babies are born only into families. Of course, many people do not follow that rule, especially in an era when sex does not automatically produce babies. But there are still restrictions on sexual behavior, and these apply especially to young people.

Your parents, your religion, your particular ethnic or cultural background and environment teach you whatever standards and values they require that you meet in your sexual behavior. Your religion may condemn most or all premarital sexual activity as a sin. Anything but the mildest boy–girl interplay may offend the moral sense of your community or your family.

Even parents without religious commitment or deep-rooted moral rules often object to their children becoming too familiar with sex at too early an age. In part, this is because they don't want their children or families marked as wrongdoers by the society within which they must live. But more important, it is often because they feel that too much intimacy too young can leave psychological and emotional scars. A person who is still emotionally a child, for instance, may be forced to grow up too fast; or by being half of a couple, a person may be cheated out of developing fully as an individual.

So no matter how natural your body's urges may be, you need to control them to one degree or another, to adapt them to the demands of the culture.

DOUBLE STANDARDS

Adapting one's sexual behavior is hard for many people. It is made even harder by what is known as the "double standard." One meaning of that phrase has been that boys and men were allowed sexual experiences that girls and women weren't. That idea was based in part on the old belief that females, or at least "nice" ones, didn't have the same kind of sexual drives as men. Those that did were made to feel ashamed. Research now indicates, however, that girls and women respond to sexual stimuli in almost exactly the same way as boys and men.

Girls also were more restricted than boys because girls could get pregnant—"get in trouble"—and boys couldn't. Today the various methods of contraception make it possible to prevent pregnancy, but one still runs into this argument for the double standard. Parents, for instance, may let a son stay out until all hours without having to account for his activities, but they make a daughter come in early and report on every minute of her evening out. They don't want her to "get in trouble." This kind of attitude may not seem fair to the daughter, but it isn't really fair to the son either. If it is wrong for a girl to get pregnant before she is married, then it is also wrong for a boy to make her pregnant. Everyone, boy or girl, needs to take responsibility for his or her behavior.

These days, our society has some other double standards. On the one hand, it decrees that sex outside of marriage is wrong; but on the other, it does little to condemn those that break that rule. Adults also proclaim that sex is bad for teen-agers while at the same time surrounding them with movies, books, music, and magazines that glorify sex and sexiness.

Against this background, it is hard to set and follow standards that are right for you. But that is exactly what you need to do. When the rules were strict and clear—"no sex before marriage," "a girl who gets pregnant is ruined for life," and the like—things were easier. There was little need to make decisions; you simply followed the rules. But now you need to make your own rules.

Sexual behavior is one of the major areas in which

you can and must really take charge of yourself by taking responsibility for what you do. For there is no way in which your parents can physically prevent you from those activities of which they disapprove. It is up to you to set your own standards. You will want to study the teachings of your religion on the subject and you will need to examine your conscience—that behavior-control mechanism built into you by your family and your community. But in the end, the final choice for what is right for you is up to you.

It is important, too, that you consider what is right for *you*, rather than let your friends carry you along with the crowd. Everyone is different, and everyone develops at a different pace. If you feel pressured, for instance, into some form of sexual activity before you really feel ready for it, you may end up with a bad experience that will stay in your mind for the rest of your life.

JUST THE FACTS

As in the case of any important decision, you need to have at your disposal as much information as possible. Here are some facts you need to know, some myths you need to forget, and some pros and cons you need to consider . . .

❧ Sexual intercourse. The genital union of two people. (The word "sex" is often used to mean "intercourse." Actually, intercourse is only one sexual activity among many, ranging from hand-holding to marriage.) Intercourse usually leads to the orgasm or climax of one or both partners. Orgasm in the male is signaled by ejaculation, the discharge of seminal fluid from the penis. Female orgasm is more difficult to describe or identify since it is not accompanied by ejaculation. But like the male climax, it is marked by the sudden release of physical tensions built up by sexual stimulation. Recent research indicates that, contrary to former beliefs, the physiological mechanism of the female orgasm is very similar to that of the male.

It is possible to have intercourse without climax. It is also possible to have climax without intercourse. (And it *is* possible, despite what some people believe, for a woman or girl to become pregnant without having reached climax.)

Our society in general disapproves of intercourse—"making love," "sleeping together," "having sex"—between teen-agers, and this is one major drawback of the activity. Violating such an important rule of our culture, community, or religion creates much mental anguish. Intercourse also leads easily to pregnancy, and it is the most common way of spreading V.D.—(see Chapter Twelve).

❧ Necking and Petting. Sexual activity between two people that does not include intercourse; often called "making out." Necking usually refers to sexual arousal by kissing, hugging, and general snuggling; petting more often implies mutual sexual stimulation—excluding intercourse—that leads to climax. Making out, especially necking, is the kind of sexual activity that parents and society tend to expect of young people. They may not publicly approve of it, but they are likely to overlook it as harmless.

The only harm that making out can cause, aside from guilt or confusion on the part of those who have been taught that it is wrong, is that it can go too far and result in intercourse for which one or both partners is unprepared. (It is also *possible*, but rare, for petting to cause pregnancy, even without intercourse, if sperm is ejaculated close to the vaginal opening.)

❧ Masturbation. Stimulation of one's own genitals to the point of climax, often accompanied by sexual fantasies. This practice was once called "self-abuse" because it was once widely believed that people who masturbated would give themselves pimples, damage their brains, and make themselves sexually unfit for life. Now it is known that masturbation does not have any of those dire consequences. (The association between masturbation and pimples probably arises from the fact that the practice or the desire to masturbate first appears strongly for many people with the approach of adolescence, which is the same time when pimples are most likely to pop out.) It was once widely believed that only boys and men masturbated; now it is realized that girls and women do, too.

Masturbation as a means toward releasing sexual tensions is safer than intercourse in the sense that it involves no other person and avoids the risk of pregnancy or V.D. Despite that safety, however, many segments of our society publicly disapprove of the practice, and it is regarded as a sin by some religions. It is interesting to note, however, that according to one recent study 92 percent of the population masturbates at least once in a while. The guilt and shame that many young people are made to feel over masturbation is therefore misplaced. It is a common practice—of virtually every teen-aged boy and well over half the girls by some counts—and though it would not be considered healthy to devote all or most of one's time or thought to masturbation, it should be nothing to feel ashamed of.

❧ Male and female wet dreams. The experience of orgasm during sleep, called "wet dreams" because with boys or men, something in a dream stimulates ejaculation, resulting in wetness. But girls and women can have wet dreams, too, in that they can come to a climax during sleep as a result of a dream that excites them sexually.

Sometimes people of both sexes feel guilty about such dreams; some consider them a sin. But they are quite common occurrences; and there is little or no way to control them since they are created by the unconscious mind.

❧ Homosexuality. Sexual attraction toward people of one's own sex, as opposed to heterosexuality, the attraction toward the opposite sex (*homo* is Greek for "same"; *hetero* is Greek for "different"). Homosexuals (homosexual women are often called Lesbians, but the term can be applied to both men and women) prefer sexual activity with people of their own sex.

Opinions differ on why some people are homosexual in a mainly heterosexual world. Some experts feel that it may be an inborn trait; others point to one of a variety of types of child-rearing and family structure; still others feel that it results from a combination of causes. Homosexuality was once considered a disease, a mental disorder. Some people still hold this opinion, and many religions regard homosexuality as a sin. But to the psychiatric profession, homosexuality is simply one of several forms of sexual expression. It is certainly *easier* in our culture to be heterosexual than it is to be homosexual, but many true homosexuals have no choice but to follow their own drives. Sexual relations between homosexuals cannot, of course, cause pregnancy, but they can spread V.D.

Many people of both sexes feel an attraction for or have some sexual experience with a person of the same sex during early adolescence. A girl may have a crush on a woman teacher; a boy may find his gym teacher attractive. This does not mean that they are homosexuals for life. Rather, it is a common experience for many heterosexuals, and it is regarded as a normal stage in psychological development.

❧ Rape and other assaults. Rape is the forcing of some form of sexual relations on one person by another. We usually think of females being raped by males, but boys and men can suffer homosexual rape. Rape cannot be considered a form of sex. Rape is an assault, just as an attack with a knife, gun, or club would be.

Often, people who are raped are afraid, for one reason or another, to tell their families about it. Anyone who is raped should report it immediately. Medical attention is probably required, and anyone who suffers this kind of attack needs all the emotional help and support he or she can get. The rapist must be caught, too. Many police forces have special "rape squads" that are trained to handle rape victims, and many communities have "rape hotlines" that a victim can call to get support and advice. It was once common for the victim of a rape to be regarded as somehow being as bad as the attacker. That attitude is absolutely wrong, and luckily it is increasingly rare.

There are other ways, in addition to rape, in which sexually disoriented people can assault others and leave scars on the mind and the emotions. Unfortunately, young people are often the focus of this kind of deviant behavior. "Exhibitionists" may expose their genitals to them; relatives may convince them that there's nothing wrong with incest (sex between close family members); people with other sexual "perversions," or twisted sexual desires, may force them to do odd things that somehow provide sexual gratification to the pervert.

Often, as in the case of rape, young people are reluctant to report such incidents. But it is important that they be reported. The person who commits the act must be stopped before doing any more harm, perhaps to younger children who are even less able to cope with the situation than teen-agers are. And the victims need support and reassurance that nothing they did caused the act, and that such acts express sickness, not normal sex.

❧ Fantasies. Many people of all ages have sexual fantasies that seem to them perverted or weird, and this frightens them. But unless you *act* on fantasies in ways that you find disturbing, or unless the fantasy becomes so realistic that it seems to be controlling you, there is no need to worry that you are abnormal.

YOU DON'T HAVE TO BE A "MANIAC" TO BE NORMAL

As you've realized by now, sexual activity can create a lot of difficult situations. But you may find that you are worried because you are *not* interested in sex. Your friends may describe with pleasure the details of making out, and you have no desire to try it. Is there something wrong with you? NO! Give yourself time. Of course, it might be hard to be calm and reasonable about sex. Sometimes it seems that the whole world is sex-crazy. All of your friends may seem to talk and think of nothing else, while you're not really interested in it yet. It may seem that "everybody's doing it," but whether that's true or not (and it probably isn't), you aren't "everybody." You are developing at your own pace.

Many people pass through adolescence without having any sexual experiences. The drive to excel in athletics, academics, or creative arts takes the place of the sexual drive. Those healthy outlets are certainly more socially acceptable ways to release energy than any of the various forms of sexual activity.

If you are worried about any aspect of your sex life, including the lack of it, find someone to talk to. It would be good if you can talk with your parents about it, since their values and concerns are the ones you've grown up with. If you can, you're all that much nearer to forming a new, close relationship as adults and friends. And maybe you can—some parents are timid about the subject, but will open up when given the chance. But too often, discussing your sexual feelings and worries with parents can be difficult, if not impossible. Their moral beliefs may be too strict to allow such discussions. Also, in some cases parents, no matter what their moral attitudes, find it hard to accept that their children are growing up; they don't like to think about their teen-agers having sexual activities or problems, so they close off the topic of conversation.

Sex *is* hard to talk about, and for that reason alone it can cause unnecessary trouble. Your doctor or some other understanding adult can help relieve some of the worries you may have about it, and perhaps offer guidance in this first big test of your "selfhood."

6

"AM i GOiNG CRAZY?"

The changes that are going on inside and outside of your body are *not* easy to cope with. And sometimes you may feel as though you're going bananas. In most cases however, the "craziness" of adolescence is normal and understandable.

Think about it. You have pressures from school, from your social life, from your family, and from your body. Add to all that emotional ups and downs that can sometimes be alarmingly abrupt. One moment you may be joyously floating on happy clouds; the next, you feel like groaning under a weight of despair. You may fly into a rage and then wonder what could have made you so angry. You're not the only one to have these experiences. Adolescence, when you are growing up socially, intellectually, emotionally and physically, is famous for its ups and downs.

According to some theories, the extreme shifts in feeling that many adolescents experience are due to the body's adjustments to all the new hormones that are gushing through it. That explanation may be correct though there is as yet no firm evidence linking adolescent moods with the hormones of puberty.

Other experts explain that teen-agers, caught between childhood and adulthood, react and behave sometimes as children and sometimes as adults. That makes sense, too. For the first time in your life, you are really aware of your future, for instance. It can be an exciting prospect, filling you with energy and enthusiasm, but it can also be scary, making you want to be a little kid again, when you lived from day to day. You may have a lot on your mind besides your future, and according to one theory, you are now *capable* of having a lot more on your mind than you ever did before: your brain has developed sufficiently so that it can handle large concepts, and that can lead to large worries. How nice when all you had to remember was your name and address!

The world you live in may make it hard for you to decide whether you're a kid or a grown-up. Your parents may treat you like a baby, overprotecting and overrestricting you, while your teachers may demand the kind of responsibility and thought that they would ask of an adult. Your body is ready for adult functions, but the laws and customs of our culture insist that you must still live as a dependent child. No wonder you have ups and downs.

If you let yourself worry too much about your worries, you can get yourself into a funk. And it doesn't help your frame of mind to be told by the adults around you that "these are the best years of your life!" People who say that have forgotten the kinds of pressures and tensions they suffered under when they were your age, or they are so envious of your just starting out on life that they manage to ignore the drawbacks.

PROBLEMS WITH PARENTS

It may seem that your parents don't understand you. Maybe they don't: after all, if the adolescent you is a "new person" for you, it is for them, too. But sometimes it may seem that the problem is more than a simple lack of understanding.

The same people who seemed like loving, protective gods just a few years ago may now seem like stupid, tyrannical demons. You look at them now and they are full of flaws. You may decide that you hate them. That can be frightening, since these are the people on whom you used to rely the most. But these feelings, and the family fights that go with them, are also common. You are leaving childhood and growing toward your own adulthood. According to the customs of our culture, you will be leaving home soon. You would never leave if you thought it was perfect, so it is natural that you may go out of your way to find faults that you never thought about before.

Some families are able to handle this time of upheaval calmly and constructively; for others, the entire period of adolescence is an unending pain for all concerned. If conflict does occur, it is most likely to be sharpest between mothers and daughters when the girls are twelve and thirteen, and between fathers and sons when the boys are sixteen or seventeen.

You can help to keep things smooth first by realizing that such tensions are common, and then by thinking about the contributions that you make to the problem and about ways in which you can take responsibility for your own behavior. It can't all be your parents' fault; it takes two sides to make a fight. Also, many teenagers tend to see their parents' problems as worse than they are: a drink means a parent is an alchoholic, a fight means a divorce is brewing, and so forth. See if you can be more objective than most.

Of course, sometimes families have conflicts that are not just growing pains. Sometimes parents have problems that are not just in your imagination. They may be alcoholic, or violent, or terribly unhappy. It is not your responsibility to solve their problems, but you may need help in dealing with the trouble that their problems cause you. Talk to your school counselor, your doctor, or some other adult you trust, or get in touch with one of the organizations in your community that provides professional help in dealing with family problems.

HELPING YOURSELF

Many people your age show that they realize they are often partly to blame for the conflicts they find themselves involved with by asking for advice on ways to control their emotions and behavior. That kind of interest is a big first step. Once, your parents could help you to keep your cool; now it's time for you to start taking charge of yourself. And there are a number of practical ways in which you can control or redirect your emotional ups and downs. You may not be able to keep a lid on your newly intense emotions all the time; you may not be able to make your problems disappear, but you can find ways to make it easier to live with them. Some of the suggestions below may sound simpleminded, but give them a try and see if they don't help.

❧ Understand that ups and downs, conflicts with parents, and anxieties over school and social life are common at this time of life—and try to stop worrying about your worries.

❧ Get to know yourself—your moods, your likes and dislikes, your good and bad points and the reasons for them—and work at feeling good about yourself. Find something that you like to do and are good at, and concentrate on it. It might be sports, or math, or cooking, or music, or a job—anything that is *yours*. The self-confidence that you gain from doing your own thing can be a big help in getting you through the rough spots.

❧ Find outlets for your tensions and emotions. Be creative without worrying about how well you can do: pour your feelings into a painting or a story, a diary or the piano instead of letting them build up and explode.

❧ Get lots of exercise. You'll find suggestions for physical activity in chapters sixteen and seventeen. You might be surprised at how much a walk or a bike ride can do to calm your nerves or lift your spirits. The right food and sufficient rest are valuable mood stabilizers, too.

❦ Take yourself away from a bad scene. If you feel that you are about to explode, go to your room or take a walk and give yourself time to calm down. If a situation at home is becoming unbearably tense, visit a friend or go to the movies. If you don't have be personally involved in some conflict, don't get yourself involved; leave others to their own hassles.

This does *not* mean run away from home. Too many teen-agers, unable to cope with their families or the problems of their daily lives, think that breaking loose completely is the best escape (and one that will punish their parents, as well). Then they find themselves in a strange place with no money, no chance for a job, and easy prey to people who exploit them. This kind of "solution" is worse than the problem, and the runaways are the ones who end up being punished.

Even at its best, running away is only a temporary escape, because you are not Peter Pan; you do have to grow up, no matter how painful the process may seem sometimes. By running away, you only temporarily postpone the unavoidable. Better to face up to it now and get it over with.

If a particular situation at home does make it seem impossible for you to live there, perhaps there is some place else you could go. You might live with a grandparent, a sibling, or some other relative, for instance. If you think that a move would help, get counseling, think it through, take charge of yourself and do it right—or risk making your life even more unbearable.

❦ Communicate. If you do have a problem with your parents, or with anyone, try to talk with them about it. If you can't do that, talk to *someone*. Your friends can often provide support, and one of the reasons that most teen-agers surround themselves with a large group of people their own age is to ease the transition from their home-centered childhoods toward their adult independence. But sometimes your friends can be too close to a situation, or too wrapped up in their own problems to be of real help, and you need to look for a fresh ear. Members of the clergy are traditionally good listeners; your doctor should be. Or, you may have a favorite teacher or coach, a neighbor, a relative—there is probably someone in your life whom you trust and who has the experience to understand whatever it is that's bugging you. Also, many communities have walk-in centers or telephone hotlines for kids who want to get advice or let off steam. Maybe these friends and professionals can solve your problem, maybe not—but just getting your worries out in the open is often enough to make them go away.

YOU ARE NOT ALONE

The ups and downs, the conflicts and tensions of the teen years can be very distressing. It is important to remember that you are not the only one going through these experiences; they are common and in most cases quite understandable.

But for some young people, the fears and pressures go far beyond the range of normal and cause them to sink into deep depressions, explode in wildly hostile behavior, or attempt suicide.

Suicide is the second most frequent cause of death for people aged fifteen to twenty-four, and the suicide rate for both ten- to fourteen-year-olds and fifteen- to nineteen-year-olds rose sharply in the early 1970s. That's scary, isn't it? And it doesn't include those young people who unconsciously kill themselves with drug use or "accidents." It's even scarier when suicide or thoughts of it come closer than statistics—when you or a friend of yours feels down enough to want to die.

What often gives people the final incentive to kill themselves is the feeling that they are absolutely help-less to solve their problems and that they are absolutely alone. They may be cut off from their families, deserted by their friends—but they are not alone. Help is avail-able. If you ever consider the idea of suicide, or if a friend seems likely to attempt it, get in touch with your local suicide-prevention bureau, suicide hotline, hos-pital emergency room, or rescue squad.

SIGNS OF INSANITY

A number of people your age ask to learn the symp-toms of mental illness, perhaps in part because they are afraid of becoming mentally ill themselves. It would be impossible, and not particularly helpful, to try to list all the symptoms of mental illness. Mental illness is not a single disease, like measles; there are many types and degrees of emotional and psychiatric problems, and psychiatrists don't even know all the symptoms or the causes.

You might assume that a guy who walked around talking to himself, or a girl who dressed herself up in weird clothes all the time was nuts, but you would not necessarily be right. People can appear to be perfectly normal and at the same time have things going on in their minds that are completely separating them from reality. Extreme fatigue, sleeplessness, persistent blues or loss of appetite, far-out fantasies that are more than occasional daydreams, uncontrollable emotional out-bursts or urges—any emotion or behavior that is odd for you and lasts for a while, all these can be signs of mental illness; but they can also be symptoms of a number of other problems, major and minor.

Only you know what's going on in your own head. The best advice for anyone who fears that he or she is becoming mentally ill is to see a doctor and discuss the suspected symptoms. You are probably *not* going crazy. But it is far better to talk with a professional about the symptoms that concern you than to worry about them, no matter what they are.

7

"but i feel sick!"

Have you ever gone to the doctor for a stomachache, a headache, a rash, or some other symptom and been told that there's nothing wrong with you? Many of our aches and pains have no physical cause, but that does not make them any less real or uncomfortable. Still, how is it possible to have a stomachache when there's nothing wrong with your stomach?

IS IT ALL IN YOUR MIND?

Doctors don't fully understand the connections between emotions and physical conditions. There are few ways to study these connections scientifically, but we and the doctors know from experience that the connections do exist.

Think of the phrases we commonly use. We say "up-tight" to mean that a person is tense and overly concerned with things that shouldn't matter. People who are uptight tend to hold their bodies tightly, too: their muscles are tense, their hands may be clenched, their jaws clamped firmly together. When we advise someone to "hang loose," we mean relax, take it easy, be flexible. Someone with that mental attitude also has a body that's loose, whose muscles and joints aren't locked into tense, rigid positions.

When you "sweat over" studying for an exam that turns out to be "no sweat," you can "breathe easier." You may not be thinking in physical terms, but that's what you are saying: You get so nervous about the exam in advance that you raise your body temperature enough to cause your sweat glands to cool you off with perspiration, but when you discover that the exam doesn't make you so nervous, the knots of tension in your chest loosen to allow you to take a good deep breath and really relax.

Phrases like those express the interrelationships among our moods, our mental states, and our physical condition. Because this is such a common human experience, you can probably think of many more.

How about a problem that's a "headache" or a situation that makes you "sick to your stomach"? Worries and emotional pressures *can* cause headaches, as the emotional tension is converted into physical tension within the tiny nerves and blood vessels that serve the brain. A stomach operated by muscles that are too tense won't work properly, resulting in indigestion, nausea, or "heartburn." Intestinal muscles that are too tense can cause constipation; those that are overactive when the body is in a nervous state can lead to diarrhea.

Doctors refer to tension headaches or nervous stomachs as "psychosomatic" illnesses. *Psyche* is the Greek word for mind; *soma* means body; together they make a word meaning a physical problem caused by an emotional or mental state. The headache or the stomachache is not just in your imagination; it is very real and feelable, but it is not caused by any physical disorder such as a cold or the flu.

Of course headaches, stomachaches, or any other unhealthy symptoms are not always psychosomatic. They may indicate real physical problems. If you have a severe or persistent abnormal condition—one that hurts a lot or that lasts for more than a few days—don't just assume it's "nerves," see a doctor. The doctor will check for all the possible physical sources for the trouble before concluding that there is none.

And then what happens? A psychosomatic disease can't be "cured" with medication, though aspirin or bicarbonate of soda or some other drug might ease the pain. But the problem won't go away until the cause is removed. That is when a good doctor will spend time talking with a patient, to find out if trouble at home might be making daily living a headache, or if pressure to do well in school has tied the stomach in knots. Then the doctor might suggest ways to ease the external stress and calm the body down. Or perhaps only time can cure the ailment. Sometimes just understanding the cause of the problem is enough to make the symptoms go away, for just as the mind caused the pain, so the mind can make it disappear.

Although, to repeat, any persistent physical problem should be checked thoroughly by a doctor, there are some ailments, like ulcers, headaches, and certain allergies, that are frequently psychosomatic in origin. But sometimes the "psyche" can be quite ingenious in affecting the "soma." Take a guy who wants to spend time stamp-collecting but whose father wants him to make the football team. He can't say no to his dad, but he might quite by "accident" break an arm and get off the hook. A little girl's parents may send her to summer camp against her will, and then she develops such an allergy to trees that she has to come home. A person who's feeling left out may develop a cough that attracts the attention of everyone in the room. Someone who's feeling terribly sad or depressed but won't admit it may come down with an unusual number of colds, for those watery eyes and sniffles are a lot like weeping.

None of this behavior would be conscious. The boy wouldn't decide to break his arm; the girl wouldn't will herself to get allergic to trees; no one would think "If I keep coughing they'll have to pay attention," or "I can't allow myself to cry, but I can catch cold." These people may not even realize that they're feeling tense, worried, ignored, or sad. But those feelings are there, and they need to find some outlet. If the person won't express them directly the body will. How the body handles the situation varies from person to person.

The field of psychosomatic medicine is relatively new and science has not yet thoroughly explored the mechanisms by which worries, fears, depressions, or other psychological states can throw the body's internal involuntary network of nerves, smooth muscles, and hormone production out of balance.

DISPLACEMENT AND DIS-EASE

But one thing that doctors who work with teen-agers say about their patients is that adolescents worry too much about their bodies. A boy may come into an adolescent clinic terribly upset about his "awful" case of acne, when all he has is a few pimples on his chin. A girl may be frightened by the "fact" that her breasts are the "wrong shape," when they are perfectly normal. So why are these kids worried?

Well, they're not really worried about their zits or their tits, though they may think they are. They're worried about school, or about getting along with their parents, or about too little or too much dating, or about just plain growing up. But it's a lot easier to worry about their bodies, so they "displace" their problems by focusing on something that's simpler to deal with than the real worry.

People of all ages express their personalities, their moods, and their troubles through their bodies in one way or another, but this phenomenon is especially common among teen-agers. As one adolescent specialist puts it, most of her patients are not suffering from disease, but from dis-ease. That is, they are not at ease with their bodies or with their lives, and this situation causes physical discomfort.

Also, because teen-agers may be aware of their bodies for the first time, and because they may have the first inkling that they won't live forever, problems tend to become enlarged. A mole that you have always had but never paid attention to suddenly "becomes" skin cancer; a strained chest muscle is imagined to be a heart attack.

It's perfectly understandable; after all, your whole life is changing very rapidly, and it takes a while to get used to the new you. School, family, friends, and your body itself have all become sources of new kinds of pressures, stresses, and strains. It's natural to react to that kind of pressure, and your body finds ways of doing it if you don't.

WORRYING YOURSELF SICK

A lot of people worry themselves sick by worrying about being sick. For example, a boy may be convinced that his headaches are caused by a brain tumor, and he may worry himself into worse headaches by brooding about the imaginary disease. A girl may be so afraid of getting menstrual cramps that she ties her insides into knots and really cramps up. Acne may seem like such a serious problem to some people that their worries about it make them feel sick. Or a girl may miss a menstrual period (a common occurrence among young teens) and become so convinced that she has somehow gotten pregnant that she starts getting "morning sickness." A budding athlete may decide that the pains in his feet (caused by the wrong-sized shoe) mean that he's a cripple, and avoid trying out for the track team.

Worries like these may sound silly when they're put down on paper, but when they are in your head they are not at all silly, and they *can* make you feel sick. The simplest and best thing to do whenever you have a worry about your health, no matter how silly you think it might sound, is to ask your doctor about it. An examination can show that you haven't a brain tumor, that you aren't pregnant or crippled. A prescription can help clear up the acne and ease the cramps—and then you have one less thing to worry about.

WORKING IT OUT

Medicine may not be able to cure psychosomatic ailments, but there are other ways to handle them. If you have a persistent unusual symptom like a headache, stomachache, rash, or extreme fatigue, the first thing to do is see the doctor and find out if there is a physical cause for it. If there isn't, you might be told that it is "just nerves" or "tension" or "growing pains."

You might think that a tranquilizer or pep pill would be the solution, and try to talk your doctor into prescribing one. A wise doctor, however, would be extremely wary of popping drugs into teen-agers except in very special cases. Not only is it not a good idea for anyone to rely on drugs for every down or uptight feeling, it is especially hazardous for someone of your age. Your body's balance is already tricky enough in its normal growth and development state without adding more chemicals to the confusion. Or your doctor might give you something to ease the headache, soothe the stomach, or stop the itch—and that might help the symptoms. But it is really up to you to solve the underlying problem.

So you think about it. What is it that is making you tense or nervous, or that weighs so heavily on your mind that getting out of bed in the morning is a struggle? Is it a specific problem? A fight with a friend, exams coming up, too many or not enough after-school activities? Is it a more general difficult situation— family trouble, pressures from school, worries over your social life? Be honest with yourself and try to pinpoint the trouble as closely as you can.

Then try to solve the problem—talk out your disagreement with your friend, get help in preparing for the exams, cut down or add to your social activities. If you've got troubles you can't really deal with, find someone with whom you can talk about your parents' fighting or whatever. Get your worries off your chest and they'll leave your gut and your head, too.

In the meantime, be nice to yourself. Break your routine and give yourself a treat like buying something you've been wanting or going someplace you've been wanting to. And try getting extra exercise. It's amazing how a long walk or bike ride or swim can cure a sour stomach. Why? Who knows? Again, the words we use might offer a clue: we talk about "working out" a problem, and when we exercise, we "work out." For whatever reasons, a workout of some sort often helps to work the tensions and worries out of your system.

8

"i caN't sleep!"
aNd otheR headaches

People your age indeed have a lot on their minds, a lot of new feelings to cope with. Since your mind and your feelings are part of your body, your worries and your emotions often can express themselves through your body. Sometimes these physical symptoms of "nerves" or tension can be quite troublesome. But they are not difficult to deal with once you see them as symptoms or signs of trouble rather than as problems or diseases in themselves.

THOSE SLEEPLESS NIGHTS

Insomnia, or the inability to sleep, can be a terrible, uncomfortable, and disabling condition if it persists. You have probably found that the night before an exam, a big game, a school performance or the like, when you know you ought to get a good night's sleep, you can't. Your notes, your strategy, or your lines keep running through your head. Your tension and emotional excitement prevent your muscles from relaxing into sleep. After a while, you begin worrying about not being able to sleep, and this only adds to your tension and wakefulness. So by the time you drag yourself out of bed the next morning, sore-eyed and headachy, your mind is more on the fact that you slept too little than on the exam or whatever.

Everybody has nights like that now and then, usually before facing some big event in their lives. But sometimes, some people are unable to get enough sleep for nights and months of nights on end. It makes their lives miserable and makes even small problems seem overwhelming. The cause of such insomnia is usually the same as that for the pre-exam sleepless night: something in people's minds or moods keeps their bodies from relaxing and letting go. The pattern is similar, too: after a period of sleeplessness, they begin to think only about getting to sleep, and day and night this worry only increases their tension.

If you find during some period in your life that you have trouble falling asleep, or if you wake in the wee small hours and cannot fall back to sleep easily, it probably means that you have something on your mind that's bothering you. Instead of getting yourself uptight about not sleeping, you're better off spending your sleepless hours trying to unearth the cause of the insomnia—tension at home? trouble at school? what? If you can solve that problem or resolve that conflict, your insomnia—the symptom of the underlying cause—will take care of itself.

If insomnia, like any other symptom, persists or is severe, you should seek professional help. But there are many techniques that you yourself can try that can help you sleep. Stay away from sleeping pills! Even the kind sold without a prescription are not meant to be taken often and they can be dangerous. If your sleeping place is noisy, if you share it with someone who can't be quiet, or if your family tends to be awake when you want to sleep, try earplugs (there's a soft, wax-and-cotton type on the market, or try big wads of cotton—just be sure they're big enough not to get lost in your ears). Earplugs drive some people crazy, but others swear by them. They may be worth a try as one very simple solution to the sleep problem.

And remember that caffeine—a stimulant found in coffee, tea, cocoa, and cola drinks—tends to keep many people awake. Cutting down on your intake of those beverages may be all that's needed. Amphetamines and other "uppers" keep you awake, too. And overintake of alcohol can cause you to wake in the predawn hours, after you have slept off the depressant effects.

It can also help to tire yourself out and loosen up your muscles with some non-intense exercise like a walk or a short run late in the day. Or try some of these relaxing exercises. They are good for getting the tensions out of your muscles before you go to bed or when you find you can't fall asleep.

Sit cross-legged on the floor, your hands in your lap.

Close your eyes and let your chin and shoulders droop. Slowly move your head back and forth, then around in a circle. Think about all those knotted muscles in your neck and shoulders untying themselves. Then, very slowly straighten up, thinking about bones and muscles falling into place. Arch your back and lean your head backward. Slowly move your head from side to side. Then slump again and repeat.

Get on your hands and knees, with your face parallel to the floor. Close your eyes. Slowly tighten your stomach muscles until you've sucked in your gut so far that your back and neck are curving upward and your chin has moved toward your chest. Then very slowly move the other way until your belly is hanging down, your spine and neck are arched downward and your chin is pointing out. Repeat very slowly, trying to feel every muscle and bone and joint shift from one position to the next.

Sit on the floor with your legs straight out, your feet in front of you and close together. Close your eyes. Curve your back and reach your hands toward your toes—the closer you can come to putting your nose to your knees, the better. Then very slowly lower your head backwards to the floor in a curving motion and at the same time curl your knees up and over until your shoulders are on the floor and your feet are stretched as far as they can beyond your head. Hold that position for a moment and breathe quietly, concentrating on letting every bit of tightness go out of your body. Then bend your knees, and slowly, keeping your back curved, bring yourself back to your starting position. It is important that you keep your back curved during the whole exercise—feel each piece of your spine move along the floor. You may not be able to get very far in either direction at first; but even if you can't, you should be able to feel yourself quite literally unwind.

A hot bath or a cup of warm milk before bedtime may help too. (But watch out that you don't make such a production of preparing for sleep that you make the problem worse.)

In bed, after you've turned out the light, you can help your body relax by clenching every muscle you have as tight as you can and then letting go. Do it once or twice with your whole body. Then go part by part: starting with the muscles in one foot, tighten them as hard as you can and then let them go as limp as you can; clench and relax every muscle you can find, all the way up to your head (you may think that you're relaxed and actually be holding your jaws tight together and squeezing your eyelids shut—instead, just let them find their natural position). Breathe as deeply as you can, so that you feel as though you're exhaling clear out to your toes and fingertips.

It's hard to keep your mind a blank, so instead, focus it on something soothing. Imagine a feather floating down in front of a dark curtain, or a cloud drifting across the sky; see the feather or the cloud in your mind and pay attention to it; think about it and make yourself feel the way it does. Or see a nonsense word in your mind's eye and look at it, listen to its sound over and over again. Or listen to your breathing and concentrate on counting your breaths: one for inhale, two for exhale; or count your breaths in sequence for as long as you can. You may find other techniques that work for you; the idea is simply to relax your muscles and clear your head so that sleep can take over your mind and your body.

One of the best ways to fight insomnia is to give up fighting it. If you can't sleep or think you can't, don't try. Turn on the light and read a book, listen to the radio, play solitaire, or work a puzzle. If there's some special project on your mind, work on it—at least your wakefulness can be productive.

Of course, your sleeplessness may not have any hidden emotional cause. Your body may simply have an internal clock, or a pattern of sleeping and wakefulness, that differs from the standard "eight hours from eleven to seven" rule. If you have trouble sleeping at night, pay attention to your body clock. What time of the day or night do you feel the most energetic? the most tired? If you decide that you are a "night person," someone who is at top form at night rather than in the daytime, you still have the practical problem of having to be up and alert for school in the morning. But you might do better to find time for a nap in the afternoon and stay up late than to try to force your body to sleep at a time when it doesn't want to.

On the average, teen-agers should get about eight hours of sleep out of every twenty-four hours. (If that sounds like a lot, remember that your body is doing a lot of growing and reorganizing, so it needs rest to keep it working as well as growing.)

Individuals' requirements for rest vary, and your sleep pattern may not be typical; but the need for sleep is something that your body will tell you about. Usually, you can't help but pay attention to its message: when you get tired enough, it is practically impossible not to fall asleep.

What sleep consists of and how people fall asleep is still something of a mystery to scientific researchers, but it is known that sleep is one of the most sensitive indicators of your emotional and mental state, and if you have trouble sleeping, it probably means that something in your life is not quite right.

WHO ME? UPTIGHT?

Your body has other ways of telling you that something is not right with your mood or your mind.

🖐 Nervous stomachs. Some people habitually "take it in the gut": their worries express themselves through persistent indigestion, constipation, or diarrhea. Have your doctor check for any physical cause for these symptoms. If there is none, try to figure out what is going on in your life that is tying your stomach into knots. While you're unraveling those problems, follow the doctor's advice about whatever diet or medicine might help relieve the symptoms and concentrate on loosening up your uptight stomach.

General exercise helps, as does taking a few good deep breaths whenever you feel your gut start to clench. Try to focus mentally on the troublesome part of your body—some people seem to be able to will their insides into shape, and maybe you can, too. If your stomach hurts, for instance, sit or lie quietly in a private place.

Close your eyes. Try to mentally locate the problem spot and see if you can't "untie" the knot there. It may sound far-out, but if your mind has caused the problem, perhaps your mind can solve it.

❧ Headaches. As you know from the aspirin commercials on TV, headaches, too, can be caused by tension. Headaches that are severe or that persist for more than a few days should be investigated thoroughly by a doctor. You may need glasses or you may have sinus trouble or some other easily remedied disorder. Some girls and women have headaches just before their menstrual periods due to a buildup of fluid, and this condition is easily corrected.

If there's no physical cause for the headaches, try the same approach as outlined for insomnia or nervous stomachs: think about the possible causes for tension and work on them rather than on the headaches themselves. In addition, try this for "fast fast fast relief." First pinpoint the location of the pain (is it in your forehead? temples? the back of the head? the crown?). With your fingers, gently but firmly press that point a few times; massage it; concentrate on relaxing your head, you'll probably find that you don't even need an aspirin.

❧ Other signals. A feeling of extreme fatigue even when you've been eating and sleeping right; a sudden shift in your appetite, making you feel hungry all the time or never hungry at all; a tightness in your chest that makes you feel as though you can't breathe; an unusually frequent need to urinate—these can be symptoms of physical disorders and should be checked by a doctor. But they are also common signs of tension or emotional conflict.

Instead of giving in to the fatigue, or gorging or starving yourself, or panicking about your shortness of breath, remember that these are symptoms, and try to find and deal with their cause.

Sometimes you may not even know or want to admit that something is bothering you, but your body will let you know. If you're not sleeping, or are constantly exhausted, or filled with aches and pains for which there is no physical cause, it may be that your body is telling you that you are under a lot of stress.

That's perfectly understandable: you and most people your age have a lot of situations in your life that cause stress. What happens to one part of your body, mind, or mood is bound to affect the rest of you. The solution can be as simple as getting in touch with your body and working with it rather than against it.

9

ACNE, b.o., dandruff, braces, and other fates worse than death

It isn't fair. Just when you really begin to care about how you look, you get acne, braces, dandruff, body odor, and other afflictions that seem to many people your age like fates worse than death.

ACNE

The zits, dots, pimples, spots, whiteheads, and black-heads that characterize the condition called acne are caused by little wads of dead skin cells, bacteria, and fatty acids that clog hair follicles (the tiny holes through which hair grows). These little balls of gunk sometimes expand beneath the skin, eating away and infecting the cells around them and producing a red, painful pocket of pus.

It was once thought that eating rich, fatty foods such

as chocolate, butter, and french fries caused or contributed to acne. New evidence suggests, however, that this is not the case. Researchers now believe that the culprit is androgen, one of the sex hormones that the body first begins to produce in adolescence. (Androgen is a "male" hormone, but remember that all bodies, no matter what the sex, contain both "maleness" and "femaleness.") The androgen stimulates the sebaceous or oil glands around the hair follicles to produce increased amounts of sebum, a greasy stuff whose purpose is to lightly lubricate the skin and hair.

But if sebum comes in contact with the germ that causes acne, it releases fatty acids that mix with dead cells to form those bumps. So, much as you may wish that you could have had acne when you were a little kid, you had to wait until your body was mature enough to produce an adult hormone. That's all well and good—but what can you do about it? For one thing, you can learn to live with it. Most people eventually grow out of acne after a few years, when their hormone systems settle down and don't overstimulate the production of excess oil.

Doctors used to think that eliminating rich foods from the diet would help acne, but since rich foods do not now seem to be the cause, skipping them can't be the cure. It used to be thought that scrubbing the skin and hair vigorously and often with special soaps and brushes was good for acne. Now it is doubted that medicated soaps have any effect on the acne germ, and doctors feel that too much scrubbing can make the problem worse by irritating the blackheads and whiteheads and turning them into big pimples.

Doctors have found that an ointment called Tretinoin, containing a substance similar to Vitamin A, is, for some unknown reason, often quite effective in controlling acne. This does *not* mean that Vitamin A pills will cure acne. In other cases, doctors are turning to antibiotic drugs taken internally or applied to the skin to kill the acne germ. Such antibiotics are usually safe but you should ask your doctor about ways to avoid possible side effects. Some doctors and researchers recommend for girls the use of the female hormone estrogen, usually in the form of birth-control pills, which counters the male androgen and has the effect of reducing the skin's output of oil. But taking hormones can be dangerous for teen-agers who are still growing. So, if your doctor recommends the use of such hormone treatments, find out why he or she prefers them to a safer course. The point is that it is now possible to cure or alleviate even the most painful cases of acne, and you should ask your doctor about the new methods of treatment.

And what about all those creams, salves, and cleansers that you see so many ads for and spend so much money on? They may have an effect on acne, and they may not. Many of the creams contain ingredients that shorten the time an inflamed pimple takes to heal, and many also hide the redness. Other remedies dry the skin and so may keep oil from building up. Neither type is harmful, if used according to instructions, and either may be helpful in easing the symptoms of acne; but neither type can cure the condition—you need a doctor's help for that.

There are things you can do on your own to prevent

acne or to keep a mild case from getting worse. You can keep your skin clean to help stop the growth of bacteria. Girls should avoid using foundations, powders, and other heavy makeup that could clog the follicles. And don't try to pop pimples! It is so tempting to squeeze the things and get rid of them, especially if they hurt. But if you squeeze a small pimple, you give it a better chance of becoming a big one. If you fool with a big one, you risk infecting it and ending up with a worse case that can leave a permanent scar.

The best advice is perhaps the hardest to follow: once you and your doctor have done everything you can to treat a case of acne, forget it. Just remember that countless millions of people your age have acne and hate it just as much as you do. But the acne will go away eventually—and brooding about it won't help.

BODY ODORS

Most Americans think they should be odorless. Since deodorants were first mass-marketed a few generations ago, we have been taught by the advertising media that it is a sin worse than blasphemy to "offend" others with our natural aromas. Now we can buy underarm deodorants, breath deodorants, genital deodorants, foot deodorants, and multipurpose deodorants that defume the entire body. We are made to feel that if we do not make use of all those smell suppressants, we should cover ourselves with shame and guilt and preferably leave the room, if not the country.

You may for the first time be aware of your body's odors for the simple reason that until recently you had almost no strong scent at all. You have always sweated, of course, because you have to perspire to maintain body temperature. When your temperature rises above normal, whether because of warm surroundings, exercise, or illness, your sweat glands produce moisture which passes through your pores to your skin. When that moisture evaporates in the air, your body temperature lowers.

But when you were a child, that sweat had no smell, and now that you are older, it does. (The urine of adults, especially of adult males, also smells different from the urine of children, and the vaginal secretions of grown and almost-grown females also have a natural odor.) How come?

If you were a young animal—a baby deer, for example—your mother would have to leave you unprotected when she went in search of food. Her instincts would help her hide you in a spot where your special body coloring would make you almost invisible. But if you gave off an odor, a predator could sniff you out and eat you up while she was gone. And if your excretions gave off an odor before you had the control to deposit them in secret places, an enemy could track you down by following them. So it is best, according to nature, for babies and young animals to be smell-less. Then when you were grown, nature would "want" you to be able to let others of your species know that you were nearby and capable of reproducing, and your adult odors would be part of that signaling system.

Okay, so it's perfectly natural to smell like a grown-up. But that doesn't mean you want to. Your odors may be perfectly normal, but if you were the only person in the room giving off human aromas you would feel uncomfortable just as if you were the only person at a picnic wearing a tuxedo. To avoid such embarrassment, there's nothing wrong with using a deodorant.

Some words of caution are necessary, however. Deodorants are not meant to be cover-ups. They are not meant to take the place of cleanliness, for one thing. If the body is not clean, it is going to smell bad because of the bacteria that are active in it and on it. No matter what the ads may want you to think, the deodorants are not wonderworkers. They will keep the body smelling for a while the way it did when it was first cleaned, if they are used on a clean body. So wash!

Also, even though an undeodorized mature body will normally have an odor no matter how clean it is, other strong persistent odors are not necessarily normal. If you use deodorants to cover up those smells, you may be hiding symptoms of a physical problem that could be treated.

If you have continually bad breath, for instance, even though you clean your teeth and use "breath sweeteners," you may have an infection in the mouth or a disorder of the digestive or respiratory system. Your breath will not be "sweet" until those problems are cleared up, and too-frequent use of many common mouthwashes can do more harm than good.

Vaginal odor is something that advertising has made people overly conscious of. Beginning in early adolescence a certain amount of odor in the vaginal area is normal, and women who try to eliminate it by the overuse of vaginal deodorants or douches can cause irritation and other more serious problems. "Feminine hygiene sprays" should *not* be used by teen-agers, as they are a prime cause of vaginal disorders. If a girl washes herself daily, being especially thorough after her menstrual period, she shouldn't feel the need to use a feminine hygiene spray. However, a strong vaginal odor that persists despite cleanliness is often the sign of an internal problem. It may or may not be accompanied by some kind of discharge (which is also not a normal condition) and should be checked by a doctor, not covered up by perfume.

Some people are so overcome by embarrassment about their own or another's B.O. that they wish they could die. Body odor isn't really worth getting so up-tight about, and advertising is the main reason that we are so embarrassed about it that we don't really know what we do smell like. What are your characteristic odors? Do you know? You should—they're part of you, and if you're familiar with them, you'll know when they are not right. If you are healthy, a clean body and clean clothes coupled with the moderate use of an underarm deodorant is all you should need to keep you "nice to be near."

TEETH

Teeth are a pain for many people. But if you are going to look good and feel good, you need to take good care of them. That means seeing the dentist, brushing regularly, and avoiding sweets just as the ads advise. But despite what the ads say, it really doesn't make any difference what kind of toothpaste you use.

By the time you're about sixteen you should have

your full allotment of twenty-eight permanent teeth; the "wisdom teeth" or third molars, which for most people are unnecessary traces of an earlier point in human evolution, may (or may not) grow in later. Your twenty-eight or thirty-two teeth are called "permanent," of course, because they're the set that has to last you for the rest of your life. But they won't be permanent unless you take care of them. The thought of losing your teeth may not trouble you now; but sometime pay attention to your older relatives and see the kind of hassle they have in coping with their false teeth. Think about it.

What probably does trouble you now about your teeth, in addition to the pain of a bad tooth or aching gum, is that decaying teeth or infected gums can give you bad breath, and dirty teeth do not look nearly as attractive as clean ones. So it's worth the trouble to take care of your mouth. (By the way, if you hate your teeth because they aren't as shiny white as your favorite star's, stop fretting: models and actors usually either have caps over their natural teeth or paint them with a substance that makes them look whiter than they really are).

And then there are braces. Orthodontia (literally, "teeth straightening") causes many preteens and teenagers more social and emotional agony than almost anything else they must endure during this stage of their lives. But if your dentist recommends it, it's worth the trouble. Once the braces are off your teeth, your mouth and your whole face are going to have a lot less trouble performing the vital function of eating than if you hadn't had the braces.

The best thing to do is consider them a necessary (and temporary) evil. Remember that 2.4 million American kids wear braces. It is the in thing. And they don't look as bad as you imagine they do: they're like eyeglasses—when people first start to wear glasses, they look odd, but soon the person looks strange without them.

And there are some kids who wish they *could* have braces. If your teeth make you unhappy because they are crooked or protruding, talk with your parents and your dentist about the possibility of having them straightened. It can be an expensive process, and that may pose a problem for your family; but you may be able to work something out if you let it be known how important it is to you.

DANDRUFF AND OTHER HAIRY PROBLEMS

Dandruff is another "flaw" that advertisements have caused us to feel more embarrassed about than is necessary. Most of what we call dandruff is simply dead skin cells from the scalp combined with oil from the scalp's numerous sebaceous glands. The body discards these dead cells in a continuous process; the rest of your skin flakes off, too, as it is replaced by new cells, though it doesn't have as much oil to combine with and it is not as noticeable. Teen-agers often have more dandruff than people of other ages, because their skin is temporarily producing excess oil.

You can eliminate this type of dandruff simply by keeping your hair and scalp clean and brushed to get rid of the oily dead cells. A special dandruff shampoo is not really necessary, but be sure that, whatever you use, you rinse it out thoroughly: sometimes "dandruff" is actually flakes of dried soap that has been left in the hair.

Heavy flaking, or flaking that is accompanied by itching or the falling out of hair, is another matter. It is often a sign of a scalp or skin disorder and you should ask your doctor about it. No amount of washing with commercial dandruff shampoos will help until the underlying problem is treated medically.

Small quantities of hair fall out continuously and are replaced in the body's maintenance and renewal process. Like other animals, we shed, and you may notice more hairs in the sink in some seasons of the year than in others. If your hair seems to be falling out or breaking more than usual, it may be because you have bleached or dyed it, overused dryers or curlers, washed it too often, or gone too long without a haircut. Try leaving it alone for a while or getting a trim, and see if it recovers. If you seem to be losing large quantities, even clumps, of hair, see your doctor. Unusual hair loss can be a sign of various diseases and unhealthy conditions.

Your hair may also respond to your moods. Hair loss frequently accompanies great emotional stress or tension. And it can indicate the state of a person's general health: when people are sick, their hair is often duller or limper than when they are well. So for a bright, shiny head of hair, you may need good health and a positive frame of mind as much as the perfect shampoo.

To shave or not to shave? Most boys can't wait until they have a beard worth shaving. Most men would do almost anything rather than have to shave their faces every morning. That's the way it goes—you can't wait to grow up, and then you wish you hadn't. The best place to learn how to shave is from your father or from an older brother or friend who has been shaving for a while. If you have a bad case of acne, it might be a good idea to ask your doctor for any precautions you should take in shaving.

For girls, shaving can pose a different problem. Your mother may not shave her legs or underarms, and so may disapprove if you want to. Or current fashion may dictate that you not shave your body hair, and your smooth-skinned mother may disapprove of *that*. Whatever style you choose, there is one common myth that needs to be dispelled: after the legs are shaved, the hair that grows back is *not* coarser or thicker than the hair that came off. It may appear to be because what you feel is stubble—the first sharp prongs of hair as they poke through the skin. But once you start shaving, it's hard to stop, because the new growth is, for a while more noticeable (and in places where you rub against yourself, more uncomfortable) than the original growth.

Girls don't need any "feminine" equipment for shaving; just a sharp, clean razor, hot water, and men's shaving cream will do fine. If you use a depilatory, a chemical hair remover, be sure to follow the directions carefully. Don't let the stuff stay on your skin any longer than the label recommends. It is a powerful substance, so it's a good idea to test it on a small spot on your skin before slathering it all over. And never, never use a depilatory on your face or other delicate area of your body unless the label specifically states that it is safe for skin other than legs, and unless you have tested it first!

CRAMPS AND OTHER MONTHLY TROUBLES

An old-fashioned term for menstruation is "the curse," partly no doubt because of the pain that sometimes accompanies it. Although cramps make many women and girls uncomfortable at least occasionally, their exact cause is not known. It is clear that regular, severe pain before or during monthly periods is *not* the norm, no matter what your mother or gym teacher may tell you. Cramps do tend to be worse for teen-agers than for older women; beginning in late adolescence they may be more severe for a few years than they will be later in life. But a girl who finds herself in agony every month should see her doctor to make sure that her internal organs are structured and functioning properly. It is thought that menstrual pain is more severe during periods that follow an ovulation, (many people do not ovulate every month) and that is why, in severe cases, doctors will sometimes prescribe a birth control pill for grown women to prevent ovulation. Teen-agers who take birth-control pills before their menstrual cycle is fully regular may face long-term menstrual problems as a result.

Cramps tend to be worse if you are overtired or have been eating poorly. And if your body is in good overall shape it has less trouble with every physical condition, including menstruation.

Here are some exercises that prevent or cure cramps for many people.

When you have bad menstrual cramps, your tendency may be to tighten up your body in an effort to ward off the pain. That only makes cramps—or any kind of pain, including the agony of a dentist drilling—worse. You'll get more relief if you make a conscious effort to relax your entire body. Breathe deeply. Concentrate on relaxing and breathing; you'll find that you notice the pain less.

The "knee-chest" position is a traditional and effective way to ease abdominal cramps. Get on your knees and elbows, with your hands overlapping and one cheek resting on your hands. Draw your knees up a little so that your back is arched slightly and your fanny is sticking way up in the air. Relax all your stomach muscles so that your belly just sags. If you put a pillow under your belly and a heating pad on the pillow so that your belly is against the heat, you've got an even better "cure."

Some people find that other exercises, done regularly and *before* they have cramps, help prevent menstrual pain.

Stand sideways next to a wall. Bend the elbow near the wall and raise it to shoulder height. Position yourself so that your elbow and lower arm are resting on the wall and your body is straight. Place your feet slightly apart. Put your free hand on your outside hip, just above the thigh and slightly below the hip bone. Gently push your hips toward the wall keeping your knees straight. If you are doing it right, your hips will twist slightly and will not touch the wall. If your hip touches the wall, you're doing it wrong. If you feel a very slight stretching of the abdominal muscles as your hips "try" but fail to reach the wall, you're doing it right. Push slowly and gently, but firmly, as far as your hips will go, a few times on each side. Do it regularly when you do not have your period and you may find that you have less trouble when you do.

Another way to stretch and strengthen your abdominal muscles: Get a moderately thick book. Stand with your feet apart and the book clasped in both hands high over your head. Arms and legs straight, make a circle, down toward the floor and back up again. Do it a few times in one direction, then a few times in the other.

Remember that severe menstrual cramps are not just something that you have to endure because you are female. If they occur regularly even when you are well rested, not under a lot of emotional strain, and not on some freaky diet, you should ask your doctor about them. They may be a sign of trouble that the doctor should look for, or they may be something that the doctor can help you treat medically.

Many women say that when they're happy and feeling generally good about themselves, menstruation is less painful than when they're feeling down and dissatisfied with themselves.

Depression, irritability, water retention, indigestion, bowel disorders, headaches, and backaches are also problems that can sometimes precede menstrual periods. It is thought that these symptoms are caused by hormone shifts that the body undergoes following ovulation. They also can be connected with how you're feeling about life in general, and with how you feel about your periods. For instance, some girls are over-joyed when they first menstruate; others, especially those who don't feel that they are ready to be a grown-up, find it a frightening and depressing experience. Or, if you tend to get cramps, you may unconsciously get tense and gloomy as your period approaches because in the back of your mind you are dreading the cramps. If you can get in touch with yourself, you may be able to psych yourself out of these problems. If they are severe, your doctor may be able to help.

How you manage your periods, whether by napkin or tampon, is up to you. The use of tampons avoids the odor frequently associated with menstruation, because the discharge smells only when it comes in contact with the air. But many young girls find tampons difficult to insert, and since many napkins today are impermeated with deodorant (or you can sprinkle some baby powder on them), that, combined with careful washing, can take care of the odor problem.

Tampons may require practice, but they will *not*, despite old wives' tales, destroy your virginity.

Other myths worth ignoring. You are *not* "bleeding." Some girls, especially those who have not been well prepared for the onset of menstruation, are terrified that they are hemorrhaging internally or that their insides are falling out. The discharge consists of cells from the inner lining of the uterus that have been building up since just after your last period; when these cells separate from the uterus, they break some small blood vessels, and blood colors the discharge. You only lose about two tablespoons of blood each month, but even that amount can deplete your body's iron supply. Eat some iron-rich foods—for example, prunes, raisins and green leafy vegetables—and ask your doctor about taking an iron supplement. If you notice a bloody discharge from your vagina when you do not have your period, you should check with your doctor.

There is nothing wrong with bathing, exercising, swimming, or otherwise leading a normal life during your period. If you really feel lousy and your body resists exercise for a day or two, then listen to it and take it easy; but otherwise go on as usual.

Menstruation is a perfectly normal function, one that is going to occur for approximately the next thirty-five years' worth of months; and if you hate it, yourself, and the world every time it happens, you're going to waste a lot of your life.

Such fates worse than death as acne, dandruff, and the other faults that individuals worry about are not, of course, fatal. They need not kill you emotionally or socially, either, unless you make too much of them. A boy with braces may never smile, a girl with acne may load her face with makeup—and not only do they end up looking worse than they would if they didn't try to cover up their flaws; they call attention to exactly the problem they are trying to hide. A girl who feels that she is too tall or that her breasts are too large may slump to try to make herself look less weird. A boy who thinks his ears are too big may cover them with his hands whenever possible. And what happens? People wonder, "Why is she standing like that?" "Why is he doing that with his hands?" Then they look more closely and realize, "Oh—it's because. . . ."

It makes more sense to distract attention from your "flaws." You can accomplish this trick through careful grooming, by standing straight and walking tall, and by making the most of your personality, skills, and other good points.

Some people, of course, have physical distortions that cannot be overcome by positive thinking. A disfiguring scar or birthmark that makes people avert their eyes; a nose or a set of ears so large that they make others laugh can cause great emotional pain. And that pain can distort a person's entire life. Cosmetic surgery can correct many such disfigurements, and if you suffer because of a physical problem, even if it affects "only" your appearance, it might be worthwhile to explore the possibility of having it corrected surgically. It might change your whole outlook and personality.

But even outwardly "normal" people have parts of their bodies that they hate. When we concentrate only on those bad parts, we *can* ruin the rest of our appearance or ourselves. But if we do what we can to improve those hateful parts, and then just take what's left for granted, the flaws fall into perspective and are hidden by our good points.

What do you dislike most about yourself? What embarrasses you the most about your body? Give it some thought, and ask yourself why it bothers you so. Then do what you can to correct it, and forget about it. Whatever it is, it's only a small part of you.

10

"i HATE bEiNq fAt!"

Do you think you're fat? Before you swear off eating, ask your doctor if you actually *are* overweight for your size, age, and build. What you see as "fat" may be the early-adolescent pudginess or "puppy fat" that many teen-agers grow out of. If you've never had a weight problem and if the other members of your family tend to be slim, the doctor will probably recommend that you practice patience rather than starve yourself. This extra layer will go away soon unless you worry so much about it that you eat away at your worries by stuffing yourself.

Or your "fat" may simply be the new shape that you're growing into. A girl, for instance, who has never had "hips," may become alarmed as she watches her beam broadening into its womanly curves. Get used to that shape—you'll be seeing it for a long time. If it bulges more than you would like, try some exercises to keep it firm rather than flabby.

Or, you may not be pudgy or flabby at all, but just fatter than the TV and magazine skin-and-bones ideal. So much of our culture places a high value on being slim that it is easy to think you're fat when you're just normal. If you are feeling fat, take a good look in your mirror and talk with your doctor. You probably aren't as fat as you feel.

A word of warning even if your weight and shape are perfect: it is not a good idea to go on an unending eating binge and give no thought to your weight at all. The early teen years are a bad time to put on extra weight, because there is evidence that fat added in adolescence is very difficult to get rid of later.

FACING FAT

On the other hand, it may be true that you weigh too much. For some people, this is hard to recognize or admit, especially if their families are also overweight and they've grown up thinking of fat as normal.

You can test yourself to get an honest estimate of your weight problem. Lie on your back and place a ruler lengthwise across your waist, from your ribs to your pelvic bone. If the ruler's edges don't touch both points, you are too fat. Or try this: pinch the flesh at the back of your upper arm, at your side just above waist, or on your back just below your shoulder blade. If you can grab an inch or more between your thumb and forefinger, you have too much body fat.

Other people overestimate their overweight,

especially if they've been teased about it. They are so painfully aware of being fat that they think of themselves as heavier than they actually are, and get so upset about their weight that they eat more in an effort to make themselves feel better.

Let your doctor be the judge of how much extra weight you are carrying around and try to face yourself honestly. When you can do that, you are ready to do something about your overweight.

Fat bodies are not considered attractive in most of our society, and that may make it harder to face your fat, because in the back of your mind you may have the mistaken idea that you are wicked or stupid for being overweight. Far more important than appearance is the fact that being fat is unhealthy. Obesity can make you sick and can shorten the length of your life; get rid of that extra weight now and give yourself a chance for a longer and healthier life. At the age you are right now, overweight is bad for you because it limits the kinds of activities you can do comfortably and puts an unnecessary strain on your body. So if you lose weight, you will look better and feel better.

If you are too heavy, it is because you eat too much and exercise too little. The energy that you put into your body in the form of food is not used up in the form of activity, and that extra energy is stored in the form of fat. You lose weight by taking in less food energy and putting out more activity energy, so that your body has no energy to store and uses up the fat energy it already has stored. In other words, eat less and exercise more.

But as you know if you've ever tried dieting, it is not as easy as it sounds. For most people food is more than just something to eat; it is a symbol of many important aspects of our lives—of love, of comfort, of fun, of attention, of our babyhood when we were fed and cuddled and cared for and fed some more. As a result, we often eat not because we are hungry or need food, but because we want to make ourselves feel better, or happier or more loved. When that kind of emotional eating becomes a habit, we get fat and stay fat. And then, because we have learned that fat is ugly or that overeating is stupid, we want to punish ourselves for being ugly and stupid; and we punish ourselves how? By eating some more, so that we can suffer more from our fatness. The cycle continues and the fat expands.

So if you are going to diet successfully, it is helpful to have some idea of *why* you eat too much. Think about it. What does food mean to you? What kind of mood are you most often in when you overeat the most—are you feeling angry, lonely, depressed, excited, or what?

You also need to think honestly about how much food you actually eat. You may get your extra calories (a calorie is simply the unit used to measure energy; the amount of calories a food "contains" tells how much energy it provides for activity or storage) because your family eats large meals heavy in fats and starches. What is more likely, though, is that you get your extra storable energy in snacks. That candy bar, the soda, the bag of potato chips you swallow without thinking don't disappear, you know. Unless you use the energy they give you, they end up as body fat.

HOW NOT TO DIET

Okay, so you've faced your fat, the reasons for it, and your eating habits honestly. You've got your head together, and you decide that you are really going to lose weight. You want to get it over with soon, so maybe you give up eating altogether. That's even dumber than overeating, because you can't keep it up for long. While you're fasting, you can't properly function physically, mentally, or emotionally. And even if you lose a couple of pounds, after a very short time you're going to be so hungry and exhausted that you stuff yourself and gain it all back.

Or you may pick up a box of diet pills that promise amazing weight loss without dieting, or a magazine that's pushing a new "superdiet" consisting of grapefruit, or seaweed, or gallons of water that is "guaranteed" to take off tons in a few days. Those kinds of pills and fad diets are dangerous nonsense. Not only do they not live up to their phony promises, but they can be extremely bad for your immediate and long-term health. It is better to be fat than to make yourself sick with some crazy diet.

Some popular fad diets urge you to cut one or more type of food almost completely out of your diet. The "no-carbohydrate" system is an example of this kind of fad. So-called last chance diets would have you eliminate practically all food. People who follow other fad diets concentrate on eating a single food, like rice, grapefruit, or bananas, in an effort to lose weight fast. Such diets can be very dangerous for anyone, and especially for teen-agers whose bodies need the right balance of foods to grow well. And no-food or single-food diets are impossible to stick with for long enough to result in permanent weight loss.

The best way, the *only* way, to lose weight, stay healthy, and have the energy you need for going and growing, is to work out a diet with your doctor that fits your needs. Maybe all you'll have to do is cut out or cut down on the high-calorie between-meal junk. Maybe you can eat like your family but skip second helpings. A wise doctor will not recommend a diet that is *too* painful and difficult, because if it's too rugged, you won't be able to stick with it. And if you find that you're having trouble with the doctor's plan, say so and help to think of ways to modify it.

You won't lose weight overnight or even in a few weeks, but you will lose weight. It may require patience and self-control, but those aren't such bad habits to get into. You can speed up the pace a bit by trying out some of the more vigorous exercises suggested in chapters sixteen and seventeen; they'll help burn up some of that stored energy. And you'll find sources for other dieting and exercise information on pages 163–167. Soon you'll be feeling better, looking better, and feeling better about yourself.

CRUEL AND UNUSUAL PUNISHMENT

If some people overeat to punish themselves for being fat, others give up eating just to punish themselves or those around them. A girl of normal weight and shape may announce that she is too fat and virtually stop eating. Although she begins to look like a skeleton and barely has the energy to move, she may eat so little for such a long time that she has to be hospitalized and fed through her veins to keep her from dying.

That is obviously a silly way to "diet," and probably losing weight isn't all that's in the back of such a person's unconscious mind. Maybe she is unhappier than she can admit and wants somehow to die. Maybe she has some grudge against her parents and wants to make them suffer by suffering herself. Maybe she just wants attention.

Whatever the cause, it's likely that some powerful force in her head was driving her to deny herself life's basic need—food. Such a condition is called anorexia nervosa, but in less scientific terms it's called biting off your nose to spite your face, because there are surely more constructive ways of dealing with life's problems than starving one's self to death.

"I HATE BEING SKINNY!"

Overweight is such a problem in this country, and slimness is so highly valued, that we often forget that some people hate themselves or feel ugly because they are, or think they are, too thin.

Skinniness, like pudginess, is a stage that many people go through during their early teens. You may be growing so fast that your body puts every bit of the food energy you give it into growing, and none into padded storage. Unless you were born into a family of stringbeans, patience is again in order: you'll start to fill out once your growth slows down. You may be tempted to stuff yourself with candy and high-caloried junk foods, but that can lead to trouble if those "empty calories" take away your appetite for the foods that will give you needed nutrition as well as padding. And pay attention to what your body is doing: if you keep up your skinny-person's diet after your body shifts gears, you'll end up being a lot more padded than you wanted to be.

Of course, you may come from a long line of thin people who have always been able to burn up whatever they eat. That doesn't mean that you have to be scrawny for life. Try out some shaping and building exercises and see if they don't give you some curve and heft.

A CYCLE THAT MAKES SENSE

Skinny or fat, the important thing to remember is that you can do something about the way you look and feel, if you want to.

To want to, you have to care enough about yourself; you have to get to know the person inside that "skinny" or "fat" body and realize that no matter what you look like, or think you look like, that inside person is worth taking good care of. If you feel good about yourself, you'll take care of yourself. And the better you take care of yourself, the better you'll feel about yourself. Unlike the cycles of self-punishment, that's a cycle that makes sense. And it's up to you.

11

findinq a doctor
who's riqht for you

"Ask your doctor." That advice appears throughout this book; and it's important, for a doctor can be your best partner in the care of your body. It is also important that you have a doctor whom you *can* "ask."

WHAT YOUR DOCTOR SHOULD DO FOR YOU ....

You need to have a general physical checkup once a year to make sure that you are healthy and growing properly. Since most schools, camps, and other recreational organizations require a yearly medical exam and a statement from a doctor, it's hard not to remember to visit the doctor once a year. But the exam should consist of more than a glance and a few pokes.

It should include the doctor's asking you questions

which are particularly relevant to the life of a teen-ager. These would include inquiries about your school performance, social activities, family relationships, and use of tobacco, alcohol, and other drugs. Parts of the physical examination which are particularly important for teenagers or which are different from what they would be for a child include attention to the progress of sexual development, observation of the spine for abnormal curvature, feeling the thyroid gland for evidence of enlargement, and a blood-pressure check.

An internal (pelvic) exam should be done on any girl who is sexually active. In addition, a breast examination should be done to detect any abnormal lumps. Although abnormal growths in the breast are rare for teenagers, this is an opportunity for a doctor to teach a teenager to examine herself. Self-examination of the breast is an important habit to get into, and adolescence is the best time to learn it.

Routine laboratory tests for teen-agers are not very different from those for patients of other ages. They include a blood count, urine examination, vision and hearing tests, and a skin test for contact tuberculosis. Specific tests for venereal disease are important for anyone who is sexually active.

Okay, that's basic health care. But you need a doctor for more than routine physical treatment. For one thing, a doctor can be the best source of information on your growth and development. At this time of your life, you especially need a doctor with whom you can talk, one who will listen to you, understand you, and answer your questions about what's going on in your body.

Maybe you use a doctor who treats your whole family (an "internist" or a "general practitioner"); maybe you're still seeing the pediatrician who has cared for you since you were a baby; maybe your family uses a clinic, and you see a different doctor almost every time. Any of these systems is fine, *if* the doctor is aware of and able to handle the special medical needs of adolescents, and *if* the doctor is someone whom you can trust and who takes the time and effort to listen to your problems and answer your questions.

Too often, however, doctors seem to forget that it is *your* body they are working on. They are too busy or too bored to explain what they are doing or to consider how you feel about what is going on in your body.

If you feel that you have outgrown your pediatrician, or if you feel that the doctor your family uses doesn't give you the time or attention that you think you deserve, discuss the matter with your family and find a new doctor. There is a growing number of physicians who specialize in the field of adolescent medicine, and hospitals in many communities have youth clinics staffed with experts in teen-aged problems. Ask your friends, your local medical society, or write: The Society for Adolescent Medicine, P.O. Box 3462, Granada Hills, California 91344.

People your age need a lot of medical advice and reassurance, and you can find it if you care enough about yourself to make the effort. You need a doctor who will do more than prescribe a tranquilizer when you complain of sleeplessness or stomachaches; one who will do more than say "Stop worrying—it will go away" when you're concerned about acne. You need to be able to ask your doctor "Am I growing right?" and be answered with an explanation of what stage of development your body is at and what you can expect to happen next. You need a doctor to whom you can say something like "My little sister's breasts are already bigger than mine," or "I'm afraid my penis isn't going to get any longer," and not be made to feel silly.

. . . AND WHAT YOU SHOULD DO FOR YOUR DOCTOR

No doctor is a mind reader, and unless you say what it is that worries you, no one will know. If you don't understand why the doctor says "everything is perfectly normal" when you feel so strange, say so. If you want—or don't want—your parents in the examining room with you, tell them. Your body is more your responsibility than the doctor's and you have as much right to know what is happening to it as your parents do. But you must exercise that right and that responsibility by asking questions and expressing worries.

If the doctor says that you need an operation, or a series of tests, or the care of some specialist, ask for a detailed explanation of what you can expect. Many doctors will take a small child on a tour of a hospital or operating room before taking out tonsils. This helps to make the child more at ease. Well, you're no longer a child, but you needn't feel that you're too grown up to be fearful of medical procedures. Anybody, at any age, becomes anxious when something mysterious is going to be done to their bodies. The more you understand what is happening, the less frightened you will be.

You may find that, though doctors answer your questions honestly and give thorough explanations, you still don't understand because they've used too many technical words. Remember that doctors are so familiar with the body and accustomed to their own medical language that they may forget that their patients don't know a tibia from a fibula and may not even understand how diseases are caused. If your doctor's explanations go right through you, you can ask for a translation into nontechnical language.

Sometimes, people are afraid to ask the doctor about a problem because they are afraid of what the answer will be. A boy may find a pimple on his penis, and then be afraid to mention it to the doctor because he doesn't want to hear that he has V.D. The doctor may not even notice the tiny bump that's worrying the boy. So the boy leaves, no better off—not knowing whether he has "a social disease" or just a pimple in an odd place.

A girl may have an unusual vaginal discharge but be afraid to mention it because she's sure the doctor will recommend an internal exam and she's afraid to have one. Internal exams needn't be painful or frightening. But if your mother or a friend has described how "awful" it is, you're going to think it is awful. Hearing this or any other medical precedure described to you, perhaps by someone who has had a bad experience, will usually make it sound frightening. But if the doctor explains the procedure—how the insertion of an instrument partway into the vagina makes it possible to examine the organs in your abdomen—it becomes as "awful" as having a tongue depressor put into your mouth to permit a look at your throat.

If you ask the doctor to describe what will happen before *any* kind of examination or treatment, you will be better able to relax and make the whole procedure easier. But you can't expect the doctor to explain things automatically. If you want to know, you have to ask.

12

it can happen to you—
pregnancy and
venereal disease

One subject people your age are often unwilling to ask their doctors about, but should, is sex.

Sexual activity does have its harmful side effects, and when your body is becoming capable of such activity you should know about those hazards and their prevention and cure.

Babies are the most familiar "side effect" of sex. Once a girl begins to ovulate and a boy begins to produce sperm, the two of them together can make a baby. Having a baby at your age is not a good idea. If you aren't married, who's going to take care of it? Even if you do marry young, what kind of life are you going to have tied down at such an early age by the demands of a child? Married or not, all adolescent girls who become pregnant face the same physical dangers: the bodies of girls who conceive babies while they are still growing themselves have a hard time developing well or producing healthy infants.

Of course it isn't the health hazard posed by pregnancy that worries most unmarried teen-agers, it is the possibility of pregnancy itself. We read and hear so much these days about unmarried people having babies that we tend to think that unwed pregnancy is not a social problem anymore. It certainly is less of one than it used to be. A girl who gets pregnant before she is married is not automatically ruined for life or rushed into a "shotgun marriage." But it is still enough of a problem that kids are afraid or ashamed to tell their parents about it. A girl may beg to have an abortion without her parents' knowledge (in some places this may be illegal); she may try to hide her pregnancy somehow; or she may run away from home rather than have her family find out she is pregnant.

Any young girl who becomes pregnant and doesn't tell anyone about it is leaving herself open to trouble, for without special care during pregnancy and childbirth both the mother and the unborn child can face serious illness or even death. It is vitally important that all pregnant girls receive early, regular medical treatment. Also, a pregnancy that is allowed to go on too long cannot be aborted.

After abortion—the removal of the developing baby from the uterus—became legal in the United States in 1970, many people began to think of unwanted pregnancy as no big deal. It is true that girls and women now have more choices about when and whether to have a baby than they once did, and that legal abortions are safer than the earlier, back-alley kind were. But having an abortion is not as simple as having a tooth pulled. It can leave physical and emotional scars that are hard to get rid of. So people who think, "Well, if I get pregnant I can always have an abortion," are making a mistake by being so casual. The time to prevent a pregnancy is before it happens.

PLANNING AHEAD

Preventing pregnancy used to be very difficult. With the development of drugs that prevent conception, it is not—or it does not have to be. Contraception means taking steps against ("contra") conception, which is the union of a sperm cell with an egg cell followed by the implantation of the fertilized ovum in the uterus. (Some religions oppose contraception and abortion, but those religions also oppose premarital sex, so the time to consult one's conscience is before becoming sexually active.)

But misunderstanding and lack of knowledge make even the most sophisticated techniques useless. Too often young people rely on old wives' tales or information picked up on the street because they are afraid or unwilling to get correct advice from their doctors.

❧ Girls may borrow contraceptive pills from their friends or sneak them from their mothers' supplies in the belief that a few days' worth of pills will prevent pregnancy. It won't.

❧ Many people may believe that ovulation occurs during a menstrual period and feel that intercourse at any other time is "safe." It isn't. Ovulation occurs *approximately* two weeks before menstruation, but the timing varies widely from person to person and from month to month.

❧ Some people think that girls are sterile—incapable of producing egg cells—until they are fully grown. They aren't. Once a girl has started to menstruate, she should assume that she can become pregnant.

❧ People may do things like drink castor oil or take hot baths before or after intercourse because they think that these techniques will keep them from making babies. They won't.

The only way to avoid pregnancy is to prevent sperm from connecting with the egg cell, or to keep a fertilized egg from implanting itself in the uterus. This can be done by not having intercourse, which is the most effective method, and the way in which much of society still says people your age are supposed to handle the problem.

❧ Contraception can be accomplished by preventing the ovaries from releasing eggs, which is what birth-control pills do if they are taken according to instructions.

❧ If the ova pass through the system too fast or cannot attach to the uterus, they cannot develop. An intrauterine device (I.U.D.)—a special "coil" inserted in the uterus—performs these functions, although exactly *how* it works is not fully understood.

❧ Fertilization can also be avoided by killing the sperm cells, which is what contraceptive foams and jellies do. (However, these foams and jellies are not completely effective by themselves and should be used with other forms of contraception.)

❀ Or the path between the sperm and the egg can be blocked, as with a diaphragm or a condom. Except for condoms ("rubbers") and the less effective foams or creams, contraceptive devices cannot be purchased without a doctor's prescription, and a doctor's instructions on how to use them are vital to their effectiveness. (Using someone else's diaphragm is no good, because they come in different sizes, and if they don't fit, they don't work.) A boy may be embarrassed to buy or use condoms, a girl may be embarrassed to ask her doctor for pills or a diaphragm, but think how "embarrassed" they would be by the result of not using them.

Embarrassment is only one part of the contraception problem. Research has shown, for instance, that contraceptive pills may be dangerous for some people. Your doctor must judge whether they are safe for you. Your doctor may be reluctant to prescribe a birth-control pill for you, because if you have not attained your full growth, the hormones in the pill may interfere with normal development, and if your menstrual cycle is not yet regular, the pill can cause permanent irregularity. (On the other hand, the risks of teen-age pregnancy are so high that in some cases doctors may feel that "the Pill" is the lesser of two evils.)

Some parents may not want their children to have access to contraception or birth control information. Local laws may prevent doctors from prescribing contraception for people under a legally established age or prohibit drugstores from selling contraceptives to minors. And many boys and girls themselves have doubts about using contraceptive drugs or devices. They may be frightened by what they've heard of the dangers involved. Or they may be unwilling to plan ahead to prevent pregnancy because they do not want to admit that they would ever be in a situation where such forethought would be necessary.

Contraception may have its bad side effects socially and physically, but anyone for whom sexual intercourse is a possibility should remember that pregnancy is a worse side effect all around. Boys as well as girls need to consider the problems of contraception. A boy can't get pregnant, but he can cause as much trouble for himself as for the girl he gets "in trouble" if he is careless about contraception or if he allows his girl friend to be. Anyone who is mature enough for sexual activity needs to start being mature enough to handle the consequences.

ANTI-SOCIAL DISEASES

And anyone who participates in sexual activity has to plan ahead, not only to prevent pregnancy, but also to protect himself or herself against what used to be called "social diseases." These include the familiar venereal diseases ("venereal" is derived from the Latin word *venus*, meaning love or desire) of syphilis and gonorrhea as well as some less dangerous but still painful troubles resulting from sexual activity, both homosexual and heterosexual.

V.D. is so common among American teen-agers that health experts consider it an epidemic. This situation may be due in part to increased teen-age sexual activity, but it is also the result of the use of contraceptive drugs instead of older forms of contraception. Condoms protect both partners against infection, and contraceptive creams also kill syphilis and gonorrhea germs; but pills do not. Both diseases are extremely dangerous if allowed to run their course, but both are relatively easy to cure, especially in the early stages.

Many localities maintain V.D. clinics where teenagers can go for treatment without parental permission. But because venereal diseases can be communicated only through sexual activity (the bacteria that cause them cannot survive outside the warmth and moisture of the body) the diseases are considered shameful, and victims are too often unwilling to seek treatment.

Other ailments associated in one way or another with sexual activity are also on the increase. Herpes, a disease caused by a virus that results in sores at any place of sexual contact, is not dangerous in itself, but it can be quite painful, and recent evidence suggests that it may be linked in some way to cancer of the cervix. Various vaginal infections and fungi can be communicated or worsened by sexual intercourse, and while these are not dangerous, they can be uncomfortable and require medical attention. Body lice or "crabs" can be picked up from another person through sexual contact and also require medical treatment to kill them. (Mononucleosis was once called "the kissing disease" because it was thought to be spread only by kissing. Now it is known to have other causes.)

If you are sexually active, the best way to deal with such unpleasant and possibly dangerous side effects of sex is to be honest with your doctor so that tests for these venereal diseases are part of your regular checkups. Don't just wait until you think you have a "symptom." Gonorrhea, for instance, which is rampant among teen-agers, often has no symptoms at all, and can only be detected by simple (and painless) laboratory tests. If you do not have a doctor with whom you can be straightforward, find another doctor.

IT CAN HAPPEN TO YOU

Unfortunately, too many people have the "It can't happen to me" attitude. "I won't have sex until I'm married." "I can't get pregnant." "I won't get V.D." But it *can* happen to you, maybe not right now, but sometime.

It is estimated, for instance, that over one-half of this country's unmarried girls aged fifteen to nineteen have sexual relations fairly regularly. Fewer than one-third of those girls use contraception.

In 1977 approximately 1 million teen-age girls got pregnant, and one third of all the abortions in the country are performed on teen-aged girls.

An estimated 300,000 teen-agers are treated for syphilis or gonorrhea each year, and that figure doesn't include kids who don't know they have V.D. or are afraid to seek help.

Think about it. It's up to you what you do with your body, and it's up to you to protect it.

13

self-abuse

Does everybody your age smoke, drink, and use drugs? Of course not. But if your friends or the neighborhood big shots do it may seem that "everyone" does, and you may feel pressure to join the crowd. But misuse of drugs is truly self-abuse, and before you blindly go along with the herd, or if you are considering breaking away from it, here are some facts and arguments to keep in mind.

MIND DRUGS

The use of habit-forming or hallucinatory drugs is probably the most dramatic way in which teen-agers can abuse themselves. Drug abuse terrifies parents more than almost any other threat to their children. In part this is because many parents, having grown up before the "drug culture" was widespread, have had little direct experience in dealing with drugs; but more importantly it is because the misuse of drugs can mean disaster.

If your parents get hysterical at the very thought of your using drugs, it doesn't help you to cope with the problem. This is another important area in which you need to make your own decisions for your own good.

A drug habit can be called "self-abuse" because drugs can damage, sometimes permanently, your body and your mind. Listen—if normal changes like the increased production of testosterone can turn you upside down, imagine how infusions of foreign substances like LSD or poppy juice can upset your body's balance.

But you've probably had enough of drug-related horror tales. The following is an outline of the facts on how the most commonly abused drugs act in the human system. Take a look at it, and think about it in terms of your *own* body—the only body you've got.

❧   ❧   ❧

Psychoactive drugs are chemicals that cause a person's behavior to change by affecting one's mood, mental state, or physical senses. They operate on the central nervous system by speeding up or slowing down the pace of the chemical transmitting process that passes "messages" from neuron to neuron.

Depressants (such as alcohol, barbiturates, tranquilizers, or narcotics like heroin) slow down the nerve impulses. *Stimulants* speed them up. Amphetamines, caffeine, and nicotine, among others, are stimulants. *Hallucinogens*, including LSD and mescaline, are a form of stimulant that causes the brain to distort perceptions of reality, making things seem to look, sound, feel, or smell abnormally.

Psychoactive drugs affect different parts of the brain that control such body functions as coordination, sensual perceptions, judgment, thought, emotional feelings, and basic physiological activities like breathing and heart rate.

Dependence on psychoactive drugs occurs when a person needs to continue using them to avoid psychological or physical discomfort. Some drugs cause *physical dependence*: the body has been altered so that it requires the drug in order to function as usual. Some lead to *habituation* or "psychological dependence": the user has learned that the drug gives pleasure or relieves stress, anxiety, or tension, and fears the results of giving up the drug. Either type of dependence, or a combination of both, can be called addiction. Barbiturate and narcotic users easily become physically addicted, coffee and marijuana can create psychological dependence; nicotine and alcohol may create physical or psychological dependence (or both, or neither) according to the physical or psychological state of the individual user.

Many drugs create a *tolerance* for them in the body: to produce the results that early use of the drug achieved, increasing quantities of the drug are needed. When a drug-dependent person stops using a habitual drug, or when the effects of the latest dose are wearing off, *withdrawal* occurs: the user suffers physical, emotional, or mental distress (or all three) until the body adjusts to functioning without the drug. (Fear of withdrawal symptoms is one factor that keeps many users dependent on a drug. But withdrawal symptoms, even if severe, are only temporary.)

The hazards of the use of psychoactive drugs are many. Some can permanently damage the body. *Overdoses* of drugs, *combinations* of different drugs— including the combination of alcohol with other drugs —can kill. Since mind-altering drugs affect perceptions, mood, and judgment, they can lead to dangerously hostile or suicidal *behavior*. Almost without exception, the use of psychoactive drugs is *illegal*, for minors at least. Anyone of any age who uses hallucinogens, narcotics, or illegally obtained pills violates the law. Although the sale and use of alcohol, tobacco, and in some localities marijuana, is legal for adults, these drugs are officially banned for people under a given age. Caffeine and medically prescribed depressants or stimulants are the only drugs that are legal for use by young people—and even in these instances, "legal" does not mean "good."

❦   ❦   ❦

One problem with drugs is that some can affect different people in different ways. One guy can have a "beautiful trip" on the same acid that drives his buddy stark staring mad. And drugs, like many of the chemicals we breathe, eat, and soak up from the environment can affect people in ways that haven't been discovered yet. Do they lead to defects in the babies you may someday bear or father? Do they hamper brain development? Some studies indicate that some drugs do. The evidence for this kind of residual effect is not positive, but why make a guinea pig of yourself?

In addition to the physical harm the misuse of drugs

can inflict are the social consequences of a drug habit. Drug abuse can be regarded as a kind of social disease more damaging than the more familiar kind (and breaking a drug addiction can be a lot more painful than having some penicillin to get rid of V.D.). Drug users withdraw from the kinds of activities that are vital for a person's normal psychological and emotional development. A drug habit can cause a poor showing in school, which in itself can have a lasting bad effect. It can drain your pocketbook, too. And these drugs are illegal for teens: that means that if you get caught using or dealing in them, it won't be your parents or the principal you have to deal with, but the law.

Marijuana is considered by many to be a "safe" drug. It is an acceptable part of life among many social groups, and it has been legalized *for adults* (not minors) in some states. But marijuana is still a drug, and unlike many of the others in common use, its long-term effects are not really understood. So people who say that pot is a safe and easy high are just stringing you along. Nobody knows for sure.

"LEGAL" DRUGS

Few people get arrested for smoking cigarettes or being drunk, but nicotine and alcohol can be just as bad for you and just as habit-forming as some of the illegal drugs. Even caffeine, contained in coffee, tea, cocoa, and cola drinks, is a stimulant to which the body becomes accustomed and which it learns to "need." Nor is a daily dependence on doctor-prescribed tranquilizers or pep pills any less a drug habit just because it is legal.

All the arguments against "hard" drugs may be having an effect, because their use by young people has been declining in recent years. But there has been an increase in the use of marijuana and such "grown-up" drugs as cigarettes and alcohol. You have been raised during an antismoking era in this country. Instead of seeing cigarette ads on TV, you've seen commercials detailing the harmful effects of cigarette smoking. Despite these efforts, the number of teen-aged smokers is on the rise, with the number of girls who take up smoking showing a dramatic increase.

The earlier people start smoking, the more likely it is that they will keep smoking, and the earlier smoke-induced damage can be done. Smoking, as you may have heard too often, is linked to early and painful death from lung and other cancers, emphysema, and artery disease.

But few people your age really believe that they are going to die at all, so "early death" may still be too far away from adolescence for you to get worked up about it. Then consider the effects that smoking has right now. Irritated throats, sinus congestion, and persistent coughs all can result from smoking—it's like having a constant cold. Smoking can limit your activities in other ways as well. Smoking restricts normal breathing capacity. And that doesn't mean simply that if you want to make the track team you shouldn't smoke; the lungs pour oxygen into the entire system, and without enough oxygen, no part of the system can function at its best. So think about it.

If the good-health arguments for not smoking don't grab you, think of all the things you could buy if you didn't have to spend money on cigarettes. And "have to" is right, because once you start smoking, it's hard to stop, and you do *have to* keep buying cigarettes: they can take control of your life. The best way to quit smoking is not to start. If you do smoke, give serious thought to quitting now, before cigarettes cause any more damage to your body and before they become such an important part of your life that it's hard to give them up. For help in quitting, contact your local chapter of the American Cancer Society or write: American Cancer Society, 219 East 42nd Street, New York, New York 10017.

DOWN THE BOTTLE

Another "legal drug" that is taking control of the lives of increasing numbers of teen-agers is alcohol. Almost three-quarters of all high school students drink, and about one-third drink regularly and get drunk at least a few times a year. The average age of beginning drinkers is getting younger, and in 1975 it was 12.9 years. 1,300,000 preteens and teen-agers, or almost one-tenth of all young drinkers, have serious drinking problems in the sense that they get drunk frequently and regularly, and get into trouble as a result of their drinking.

Alcoholism is a problem, or a disease, or an addiction that is not fully understood, and many experts can't even agree on a definition for what constitutes an alcoholic. Some people seem to become physically dependent upon alcohol, as a heroin addict physically requires heroin. Others don't have a physical addiction but are so socially and emotionally dependent upon it that they might as well be addicted.

Anyone who "needs" a bottle of wine to make an afternoon bearable or an evening fun may not qualify as an alcoholic, but definitely has a problem. Anyone who can go through a six-pack of beer without feeling even slightly high, or who is moving on to "hard" liquor because beer has no effect, is showing signs of a serious problem in dealing with alcohol.

Beer and wine, by the way, are no "safer" than hard liquor. Alcohol is alcohol; hard liquor contains higher concentrations of alcohol than beer, wine or the new "light" cocktails, so it simply takes smaller quantities of liquor to cause drunkenness. You may drink "only wine," but that is still drinking. You may get drunk on "only beer," but you are still drunk.

If you feel the *need* to drink, or are simply worried about what, when, why, and how much you drink, you can get information and help from the organizations listed on page 166.

But you don't have to have a drinking problem for drinking to cause problems. Alcohol is a "foreign agent" that affects your body adversely. It doesn't stimulate the senses, but deadens them, so that nothing you feel or perceive is quite in clear focus. Perhaps more importantly, it also affects your judgment in such a sneaky way that you may not even realize that you're out of control. That side effect of drinking can be much worse than a hangover: you may feel in perfect control after a few cans of beer at a football game, and then wind up in a car accident on the way home.

In short, alcohol is just as surely a drug as heroin, cocaine and the other drugs that terrify your parents, and it is illegal, too, for young people. But the tricky thing about alcohol is that it is an acceptable "drug" in most segments of society. Avoiding alcohol completely can be difficult, and so it is important that you learn how to use it wisely while being aware of the dangers of its abuse or overuse.

ESCAPE INTO A TRAP

By the time people are your age, they are probably aware of most of the hazards of drinking, smoking, and drug abuse. They've heard so many lectures and seen so many educational films on the subject that they certainly *should* be. And yet they still abuse themselves by one or more of these bad habits. Why do they do it? Perhaps only by understanding why, can you make up your own mind to take control of your own body and life.

So why? Let's be frank: The simplest answer is that many forms of self-abuse are fun. Turning on is fun, getting high is fun, having a smoke with the gang is fun. If it weren't a pleasure, at least at first, people wouldn't do it. Few people who don't like getting high will want to do it again. But the fun is too often outweighed by the various dangers, so there must be something more going on.

What's going on in your life right now is that you're

growing away from dependence on your parents and growing toward your own independence. One way of doing that is to cut yourself off from your parents' control by refusing to do any of the things that they think are wise or good.

Some child-raising experts compare teen-agers to two-year-olds. That is not as insulting as it sounds. At two, kids are first really able to get around a bit on their own, so they want to do it—and they need to, if they are to keep growing as creatures separate from their mothers. Mommy says "no" or "don't" to a two-year-old and the little darling is apt to do exactly what she *doesn't* want, because something inside tells the kid to make some independent decisions about things.

Teen-agers are at the same kind of stage, except that they can wander farther from Mommy than into the next room. We all have to grow up, and if we're lucky we have parents who let us. One step toward growing up, whether we're two or twelve or twenty-two, is to make our own decisions. But teen-agers have an advantage over two-year-olds. If a toddler sticks his finger in a socket just because his mother says "don't," he doesn't *know* that he could electrocute his precious little self. But you know or can think about the things that you can do to yourself, and so you should be more capable of making a rational decision than a two-year-old.

The fact that your parents and teachers and the rest of the older generation—the very ones that you may feel like rebelling against—are the ones who are telling you the loudest *not* to drink, smoke, or use harmful drugs may make it harder to listen and to follow their advice. Okay, so don't listen to them. Take a look at pages 105–107 again. Take a good hard look at the people around you who do overuse legal and illegal drugs. Then use your own good sense and follow your own advice.

But even though teen-agers may know that it doesn't make sense to smoke, or drink, or take drugs, they do it anyway. And that's a sure sign that something deep and heavy is happening. Some do it to "prove themselves," to show that they're not chicken. That's like the kid who drives his car off a cliff to show how brave he is. Such physical recklessness is another common way in which teen-agers, who still don't believe that they are mortal, abuse themselves. But what does it accomplish? At that guy's funeral, everyone will say how brave he was—and how stupid. It would be braver, of course, to show that you could resist the social pressure that, in the long and perhaps the short run, is only self-destructive.

Some abuse themselves to show off in other ways. They may be very high-minded about never taking "drugs," and yet they drink alcohol for the sole purpose of getting high—so what's the difference? Or they may drink and smoke to show how "grown up" they are, though it would make a lot more sense to turn that idea around and say that drinking and smoking, like the bottle-feeding and thumbsucking they symbolize, show how childish adults are. They may take drugs to show how cool they are, but shooting heroin and sniffing glue are on the way out as fashionable things to do.

But probably that most common explanation for self-abuse is that it provides escape. As we've said and as you know, teen-agers are under a lot of new kinds of pressures. Family and school make new demands on them. Perhaps for the first time they are really aware of the problems that exist in the world, for them personally and for humankind as a whole. Their bodies keep surprising them, and they are experiencing emotions and sensations and longings that are completely new and therefore often frightening. Drugs, cigarettes, and alcohol can, if only briefly, relieve those tensions and alter that "reality." The problem is, of course, that they don't really solve any problem or change any reality, and they can cause a lot of additional problems once you're hooked.

It doesn't help to be told by the clergy that the use of that kind of escape hatch is a sin, or to hear from other "wise" adults that it is a sign of weakness. All that kind of message tells the smoker, heavy drinker, or drug addict is that he or she is a weak sinner—and how can such a weak sinner possibly find the strength to kick the habit?

More to the point is to realize that, under the circumstances, it is very tempting to look for an "escape," but that you need to be aware that what looks like an escape may actually be a trap, making you more, not less, dependent on forces outside of your own self.

You'll find ideas for more constructive methods of escape and tension relief on pages 56–64. You *can* avoid abusing yourself and entrapping yourself if you think about it and take charge of yourself and of the only body you've got. What "everybody" does or "everybody" says doesn't matter—it's *you* that counts.

14

"EATING RIGHT is boring!"

There is no easier, or more important, way of taking good care of yourself than by eating right.

You're getting to the point where you don't have to eat all of and only what your family is willing to feed you. You have freedom and pocket money with which to feed yourself, and that means you owe it to yourself to feed yourself well. Food is what keeps all your body's systems—including your brain and your emotions—going. A poor diet can make you feel sick, tired, depressed and ugly. The right food can make you stronger, more alive-looking, more energetic, and happier. It's worth a little thought about what you eat—and don't eat.

DOING WITHOUT THE THREE SQUARES

Once you realize how important proper nutrition is to you, you won't want to cheat yourself by eating poorly. But EATING RIGHT IS BORING! isn't it?

Eating right is boring because "proper diet" means three square meals a day, built around the four food groups and including liver once a week and lots of milk and leafy greens—right? *Wrong.* That ideal diet would keep you healthy, all right, but it's tedious enough to make people give up eating, and it's impractical in an age of snack foods, meals on the run, and prepackaged main dishes.

Your body, even in this modern fast-food age, still needs the right amounts of the basic nutrients in the right balance if it is to work right. But there are lots of ways to get those nutrients that aren't boring and that don't even require organized meals.

For instance, you need protein to build new cells during these high-growth years, and calcium to make the bones grow strong, but you don't have to get that nourishment from a roast-beef dinner. A piece of cheese pizza will give you one-sixth of the calcium and one-fourth of the protein that you need in a day, and a cheeseburger will provide much more. You should not skip breakfast, but you can eat a cheese sandwich and an orange on the way to school and get the same nourishment you would from eggs, toast, and juice at the breakfast table.

Check the chart on page 119 for information about what you must eat and why, and see pages 120–121 for suggestions of alternate sources for your necessary nutrition.

Remember, though, that the fact that you eat on the go doesn't mean that you can get away with eating only junk without being sorry for it sooner or later. A dough-nut and soda for breakfast, potato chips and soda for lunch, candy bars for a snack, and a hot dog and soda for dinner might fill you up, but they won't do you much good, because that kind of eating provides little of the nourishment that your body and mind need. In fact, such a diet could easily do you more harm than good because of the sugar, chemical additives, and artificial ingredients that load most processed snack foods. Nuts, popcorn, fruit, juice, ice cream, cheese, yogurt, milk shakes, pizza, and hamburgers are on-the-go foods that will do a lot more for your body (and usually your pocketbook) than the standard, highly advertised snacks. Check the chart.

FREAKING OUT ON FADS

Some kids seem to devote too much thought to what they eat. Having come to believe that the standard modern diet is wasteful, unhealthy, or immoral, they latch on to some fad by which they're going to save their souls by eating only rice, soybeans, or squid. Or they may be involved in athletics, and the coach has told them that they should eat only steak and "high energy" soft drinks, or drink no water, all in order to improve their performance.

Extreme diets that for whatever reason focus on only

MINIMUM DAILY REQUIREMENT
FOR THE AVERAGE TEEN-AGE DIET

Milk and milk products:	Four or more cups of milk or equivalent (1 cup milk = 1 cup yogurt, 1½ cups cottage cheese, 1-inch cube hard cheese or 2 cups of ice cream)
Meat, fish, poultry:	Three 3-ounce servings or equivalent (1 serving = 2 eggs, 1 cup dried beans or 4 tablespoons peanut butter)
Green and/or yellow vegetables:	Two half-cup servings
Citrus fruits and other vitamin-C sources:	Two servings (1 serving = 6 ounces citrus juice, 8 ounces tomato juice, 1 orange, ½ grapefruit, 1 medium tomato, or 2 cups lemonade)
Bread, cereals:	Four or more servings (1 serving = 1 slice bread, 1 ounce breakfast cereal or ½–¾ cup pasta)
Butter, oil, margarine:	2–4 tablespoons
Water:	32 ounces
Sweets and sugars:	None required

Source: Deutsch, Ronald M., *The Family Guide to Better Food and Health* (Des Moines: Creative Library, 1971), from the Committee on Foods and Nutrition of the American Medical Association.

ALTERNATE SOURCES FOR
NECESSARY NUTRITION

For good health, nutritionists recommend a certain number of servings a day from each of four "food groups." You can meet these requirements by eating three well-balanced meals a day, but you don't have to eat the traditional breakfast, lunch and dinner. The chart below suggests ways in which you can feed yourself properly without sitting down for a formal meal at all. Also, check the books on pages 166–68 for more information about food.

Food Group	Servings Per Day	Alternate Source
"Meat"	Three 3-ounce portions	Cheese, tuna, and peanut butter sandwiches; hamburgers, cheeseburgers; nuts. (Whole wheat bread is best for sandwiches—try some of the "soft" kinds.)
"Milk"	Four or more cups	Ice cream, milkshakes, yogurt; cheese—plain or in sandwiches, cheeseburgers, or pizza.

Food Group	Servings Per Day	Alternate Source
"Bread & Cereal"	Four or more dry ounces —whole grain or enriched	Bread in sandwiches (whole wheat is best); pizza crust.
"Fruit & Vegetable"	Four servings	Fruit juices; Fruits, especially cantalope, watermelon, bananas, oranges, and raisins. French fries, coleslaw, lettuce and tomato on sandwiches.

Note: you also need a few tablespoons of fats or oils, easily obtained through butter, margarine, or mayonnaise on sandwiches or as the cooking medium in most commercially prepared foods. Also, you should drink about four glasses of water a day. Your body needs no sweets or sugars.

one kind of food to the exclusion of others are bad for you. They can hamper your growth and they can make you sick. Your body is designed to work on a balanced interaction of different types of food, and though there are many ways to achieve "balance," you must get it somehow. If you feel the urge to be a vegetarian, fine, but learn how to get protein from foods other than meats. If you feel that your family's eating habits are wasteful of the world's food supply, you may be right. But instead of wasting yourself by eating none of it, take steps to find more economical and ecologically sound means toward a healthy diet. If you're an athlete, you probably do need to take in more calories' worth of food energy than your less active friends, but you still need a lot more than "protein foods," and you do need water.

Coaches and gurus may be expert in a lot of things, but they are not necessarily experts in the dietary needs of adolescents. It's your body, and it is up to you to see that it is well fed, not fed according to some old wives' tale or modern fad.

15

"i HATE TO EXERCISE!"

How many times during your childhood were you nagged to "go out and play in the fresh air" when all you wanted to do was sit in the dark and watch TV? You've probably always heard that exercise is good for you; but *is* it?

Human beings have been "working out" for so many centuries—whether carrying the flame in the original Olympics, or touching their toes ten times each morning—that you would think we would have some sort of scientific proof that all this effort had a purpose. Well, we don't.

It is only fairly recently that people have begun to studies have been made by gym teachers, sports enthusiasts, or others who would naturally want to show that exercise is indeed good for us. Some experts hold that exercise will help you to think better; some that it will make you more resistant to disease; others that it's important in your effort to win friends and influence people. But the studies themselves do not prove any of these claims. It is true that research has found *links* between regular, vigorous exercise and the prevention of heart and artery disease, but it has yet to show that it is the exercise itself that provides that protection.

There is measurable evidence of the immediate effects that activity has on the body. During vigorous exercise, for instance, the lungs work to capacity and the heart pounds faster, sending increased supplies of oxygen to the body's cells. Every organ and system is affected in some way by strenuous activity; in effect they are all "exercised." It makes sense to assume that this is good for us, though we don't know for sure that it is. It also makes sense to assume that the human body, like that of any other animal, having been designed by evolution to be capable of a certain amount of activity, needs that activity level to function at its best. But that cannot be stated as a fact.

It is known that exercise strengthens muscles so that the body is able to work harder and withstand more physical stress. Exercise stretches the muscles and the connective tissues so that the body is capable of a wider variety of activities. The training it provides allows the body to keep going for longer periods of time.

But do modern humans need the increased strength, flexibility, and stamina that exercise provides?

FIT FOR WHAT?

We travel in cars, trains, planes, or buses; we don't have to walk. We get our food from supermarkets, loaded into the car or delivered to our homes; we don't have to plow, harvest, or hunt. We wash our clothes in machines, prepare our food with electrical appliances, heat our homes with furnaces; we don't have to put any physical effort into scrubbing, kneading, chopping wood, or doing any of the activities necessary for daily survival. So we can be limp-muscled, lazy so-and-sos and still be physically fit for the lives we lead.

It is true that more people are dying at younger ages of heart disease and that part of the cause for this may be the low level of activity required by modern life. Also, some doctors are reporting increased cases of osteoporosis (hollow, brittle bones) and other diseases that might be traced to underactivity. It is thought that people who keep fit in their younger years are better able to be physically active further into old age.

But the only health benefit which we know for sure that exercise provides is weight control. Our easy-living modern lifestyle tends to make us fat. Though we don't have to spend much energy to survive, we don't cut down much on the amount of energy we take in as food. That unused energy is stored in the form of fat, and obesity does shorten life by contributing to such diseases as heart trouble and diabetes and by making other illnesses difficult to treat. Since exercise "burns up" that energy so that it cannot be stored as fat, it helps to prevent and cure overweight. If you had to walk five miles to school, or chop wood to cook your supper, you wouldn't have to go out of your way to get exercise; it would be built into your daily life.

But are weight control and other possible future benefits the only arguments in favor of exercise? No. They are just the only reasons for which there is any objective, scientific proof at this time. There are other reasons to exercise, but they are subjective, supported not by scientific evidence but by the personal experiences of people who do keep active.

Exercise makes you feel good. It is a good feeling to be able to walk down a street or hallway and sense that all of your body parts are working in coordination. It is a good feeling to know that you can make your body work for you, rather than against you, that you can control and direct it. It's a good feeling to know that you have some skill that you have trained yourself and your body to do well; it gives you confidence to face the other challenges of your life. Exercise can do all those things for you and more.

It makes most people feel good to know that they look good, and exercise can help you there, too. It keeps fat off and keeps the muscles in good tone. It flattens potbellies by strengthening abdominal muscles. It provides the muscular development that gives a curve to a girl's leg or a bulge to a boy's shoulders and generally gets people into the shapes that most other people find attractive.

Exercise can help you feel better physically. While it can't cure or prevent disease, it can relieve such common problems as menstrual cramps or backaches. It can loosen up tense muscles that cause the miscellaneous aches and pains that can make daily life a drag. Can you remember, when you were younger, how, after a free-for-all with your playmates, you lay gasping and giggling on the ground? Do you remember how alive and tingly you felt all over? A good workout can give you the same sensation—leave you refreshed and revitalized and, well, feeling good.

It can relieve emotional tensions, as well. Exactly why this happens isn't known for sure, but it does. As we mentioned earlier, a long walk can untie the knots in your stomach, exercise can relax you enough to sleep even when you're worried. Different tension relievers work for different people: some require a cross-country jog to clear their minds; others find that a yoga session is more effective. But it's a good bet that some form of exercise will help you to cope with your own particular tensions.

You may also find, as many have, that when your body is strong and fit you are better able to hold up under *mental* stress and emotional strain. Why? Who knows? But it's worth a try if it's going to make you feel better.

Exercise can also help you feel your "self" better. When you work your body, work with it, you get in touch with it. You become sensitive to its needs and reactions. You learn to take cues from it that warn you of tension or stress. You become aware of how it reacts to your moods and to the pressures in your life. And the more you know about it, the more comfortable you feel "inside" it. The more comfortable you feel with yourself, the better off you are.

None of these intangible benefits of exercise can be

proven scientifically. But you can prove them to your-self by finding the right kind of exercise for you.

THE WRONG KINDS OF EXERCISE

But before we suggest some of the right kinds of exercise you might try to find, you need to be aware of the hazards of the wrong kind.

Because exercise, despite its provable and unprovable benefits, can be hazardous to your health. The exact number of exercise-related injuries is not known, but in 1974 hospital emergency rooms treated about 8.5 million people for injuries caused by some form of athletics. Over one-third of those accidents involved people between the ages of five and fourteen; almost one-half happened to those between fifteen and twenty-four. To these figures must be added the injuries that went untreated or that were handled by private doctors or team coaches.

Parents may keep their children away from football or hockey for fear of the damage that these "bruising" sports could do; but other athletic activities can be equally dangerous, or more so. In the late 1960s and again in the mid-1970s there were what some have called skate-board epidemics, due to the countless injuries and even deaths resulting from the popularity of that simple-looking but difficult-to-control device.

People run their bicycles into cars, their skis into trees. They do gymnastics without proper padding and risk spine and joint injuries. They throw their shoulders and elbows out of joint playing baseball or tennis, and find that the injury, unless properly treated, returns to haunt them in later life. An exercise injury may seem minor when it happens, but unless it is treated promptly and well it can lead to later, more serious problems.

Any form of exercise can be dangerous if it is not done right. Anyone who plunges into a vigorous exercise program without working up to it gradually is going to live—or not live—to regret it. Even the fittest of people who try to make their bodies work strenuously without warming them up first run the risk of stiff muscles, dislocations, and more serious ills. And no matter how fit or well warmed up you are, you can hurt yourself by doing the right exercises in the wrong way. Many exercises designed to strengthen stomach muscles, for instance, will also injure the back if done improperly; jogging on the wrong kind of surface in the wrong kind of shoes can hurt your feet and knees.

In addition to these general dangers, mis-exercise can pose special dangers for teen-agers. Until your skeleton has stopped growing, the bones are not firmly locked together. Instead, the ends of most of them consist largely of cartilage (a softer substance than bone; the tip of your nose is cartilage). The wrong kind of stress placed on these weak connecting points can tear them. The healing process can be difficult and can often interfere with proper bone development, especially if the injury occurs during a high-growth period. Also, until the bones are long enough to act as effective levers, young bodies are not capable of exerting the strength of adults.

Another danger to would-be adolescent athletics comes from mismatching. Because teen-agers develop at such differing paces, some are physically mature at the same age that others are physically still children. Two fifteen-year-old boys may be five feet ten inches and weigh 150 pounds; but if one has gained his full bone structure and muscular development and the other is just starting his growth spurt, the first could really smear the second in any kind of competition.

You can also be mismatched for the kind of activity you are interested in. You may be dying to be a gymnast, but you have a naturally stiff body, so you face frustration at best and injury at worst if you get involved in a sport that requires so much flexibility. Or, you may long to be on the football team, but if your body is too flexible, you're making a mistake if you play against sturdy, muscular, and much less flexible types.

A series of simple tests called "S.C.A.M." (for selection, classification, age, and maturity) has been designed that will help gym teachers and coaches judge a person's physical maturity and flexibility. When these are put into wide use, they should help prevent many sports-related injuries.

Until then, you need to be the judge of your own body. Does it tend to bend easily, or is it muscular and rather stiff? Do you have more, or less, body hair than the people you might compete with? Your physical maturity and your body type will have a lot to do with the kinds of exercise that you will really enjoy.

Because, despite the hazards, the teen years are perhaps the best time in your life to get involved in some sort of exercise program. Girls in their early teens and boys in their later teens are at their lifetime's peak of physical fitness in terms of potential strength, flexibility, and trainability. Now, when it's easy, is the best time to start training your body, so that as it ages (and it will age, believe it or not) you will have less trouble keeping it in shape.

16

"How can i get into shape?"

The right kind of exercise will help you to feel better and look better. It will help you to accomplish the physical goal you set—whether that goal is reducing your hips, building your muscles, or increasing your staying power. And most importantly, the right kind of exercise is the kind that you enjoy.

If "exercise" to you has meant something like taking ten laps around the gym, or playing basketball or football against some kids who looked tough enough to murder you, then it's no wonder that you don't like the idea of exercise. But exercise comes in so many forms that it shouldn't be hard to find some that you like and can keep up for a lifetime.

THE SYSTEMS

You are probably all too familiar with the commercial exercise "systems" whose names you see on book covers in the drugstore or hear about in TV ads. They all promise to make you fit and gorgeous; they all have their drawbacks; many have advantages—and one may be right for you. The Further Reading section lists books that can give you more details on any system you find interesting.

❧ Aerobics. "Aerobic" literally means "living in air." As a fitness system it consists of a variety of very vigorous exercises designed to make the heart and lungs pump the greatest possible quantity of oxygen throughout the body. Almost any prolonged, vigorous exercise will accomplish this, since hardworking muscles consume a lot of oxygen, and the lungs and heart respond to the need by taking in and distributing large amounts of air. Aerobics, it is thought, reduce the risk of heart attack, but no firm evidence supports this claim. This kind of exercise becomes a "system" when you measure your pulse rate before and after exercise and follow a charted progression to push your body to its maximum capacity.

❧ Air Force Exercises. The United States Air Force follows the aerobic system in its fitness program. The Royal Canadian Air Force has also compiled a series of exercises, with accompanying charts and ratings. Both are supposed to work out the entire body quickly and thoroughly, and they do, but they take a lot of willpower.

❧   Isometrics. An isometric exercise is one in which the muscles are contracted tightly for a few seconds, then released. Not too long ago the isometric system was sold as a popular way of firming up the body in a few seconds a day. While it can be useful in strengthening certain muscles (and is a good way to exercise without looking or feeling as though you are), by itself it provides few overall benefits.

❧   Isotonics. An isotonic, as opposed to an isometric, exercise is one in which muscles are worked without tension. Almost any kind of activity falls into this category, but the most familiar form is calisthenics. There are at least as many calisthenic exercises as there are gym teachers in the universe. Specific calisthenics can build up or trim down particular parts of the body; a good series of them can get the whole body into shape. You can do them as part of a formal, supervised program, or at home on your own.

❧   Oriental arts. A number of exercise systems are based on the cultures or religions of the Far East. These include the "martial arts" like judo, jujitsu, and karate, and the more heavily philosophical disciplines like yoga and t'ai chi. Few of these systems provide the exhaustive workouts of the more energetic Western techniques, but done properly they can be good ways to bring your physical and your spiritual parts into harmony and to develop confidence and coordination. If you couldn't be less interested in exercise, you still might gain tremendous value from such spiritual exercise as yoga, psychocalisthenics or t'ai chi. After this type of workout, you may not feel sweaty and winded, but you can feel relaxed and energized. Some practitioners of these arts advocate special diets, designed to "purge" the body and soul. These may be extremely unbalanced, and as such can be dangerous.

❧ The schools. Commerical exercise classes have been springing up like dandelions ever since the current fitness fad took root. Some of these are based on dance movements; some use relaxation techniques; others combine calisthenics with gymnastics and yoga. Each school imposes whatever system its proprietor feels works best. Some are run by people who do have training and experience in the use and care of the human body; some are not. The advantage of such classes is that practically everyone who joins them is an amateur, so you needn't feel self-conscious about being "fat," "clumsy," or generally out of shape. Also, if you lack the willpower, knowledge, or interest to do exercises on your own, a class can force you into a routine. The disadvantages of the schools, by whatever name they go, are that they cost money (some less than others: a program at the "Y" will be cheaper than one at a fancy "salon") and if you decide you don't like it after you've signed up, you're stuck.

❧ Spas and health clubs. It's hard to avoid hearing, seeing, or reading ads for these paradises that will "reshape your body and improve your outlook in no time." They also turn a nice profit, which is the reason most of them exist. Most of them rely on various types of mechanical devices. Some of these, like pulleys or treadmills, which make the body work while it's exercised, can strengthen and shape muscles fairly quickly.

The type of machine that does nothing but shake you, massage you, or make you sweat will leave you no more fit than when you plunked your money down.

❧ Weight lifting. Body building is enjoying increasing popularity. By doing isometric exercises and lifting weights it is possible to increase the size and accentuate the shape of various muscles, and there's nothing wrong with that. But an overly developed body is not necessarily a fit body, since muscle size has little to do with health or endurance; weight lifting is by no means a "complete" exercise. Also, the diets prescribed by weight-lifting fanatics are often too unbalanced for good health. But if you are interested in developing a stronger-looking body, you might give weight lifting a try. You needn't join a gym or even invest in barbells at first. But you must use extreme caution, because a weight that is too heavy or that is lifted in the wrong way can damage muscles and ligaments.

❧ "Wonderbody in only seconds a day" programs. Almost every day a new book or article comes off the presses promising to make the reader healthy and gorgeous instantly and without effort. Some of these printed exercise programs are quite effective (though not instantaneous) if you follow the instructions. You'll find a list of the better books on page 166. Others are more interested in selling the book than in improving your body.

Into this category also fall the "do-it-yourself" devices. Every now and then the airwaves and magazine pages will be clogged with ads for some garment or mechanism that promises to make you firm and fit almost automatically. Although some of these things, like exercise bikes or jump ropes, can be useful, many of them, like inflatable rubber suits or "gravity boards" are worthless. You can set up a do-it-yourself gym at home, if you want, but you don't have to buy any special equipment and you won't get fit instantly.

WORDS TO THE WISE

Perhaps one of the systems described above appeals to you. Fine. Few can do you any harm, if you're sensible about starting slowly and not overdoing, and many will do you good. But before taking the plunge, keep these points in mind.

❧ In choosing a system, be suspicious of any that promise an instant makeover or anything close to it.

❧ Stay away from machines that "do all the work for you." If we didn't have machines that did all our work already, we would be fit without doing special exercises.

❧ If you decide to join some club, class, or organization, be sure before you or your parents pay the price that you are going to have the time and the enthusiasm to finish the course.

❧ Watch out for the special diets that accompany some systems. If you are exercising in part to lose weight, get a diet from your doctor that cuts calories without throwing you off balance. Any other kind is unnecessary and possibly dangerous.

❧ If you have a medical or physical problem, check with your doctor before beginning any exercise program. Many spas and schools require a physician's certificate, and it's a good idea for any system you choose.

❧ Follow instructions! Don't try the hardest series in the exercise book until you are comfortable with the easier stages. Your body is young and fairly limber, but you can still strain it by overdoing.

❧ Remember that many of the systems are sold, whether as books or as programs, more to make money than to improve your body, so it is a good idea to check out their reliability and usefulness before you make any major investment of time or money.

17

RuNNiNq, jumpiNq, ANd sTANdiNq sTill

You needn't spend any money or join any classes to get the exercise that will keep you feeling good. There are many ways to get in shape without following someone else's system.

SPORTS

Athletics have always been one of the most common ways of getting exercise. Athletic competition has often been the main purpose of exercise: people work out to train their bodies so that they can play and win games. But for many people, the competition of sports is a turnoff. There have always been some kids who are good at baseball, soccer, racing, tag, or whatever—any game they play, they win. The kids who have trouble winning, whether because they haven't been taught the game, or have immature bodies, or come from families where sports were not valued, eventually give up trying.

When the teachers, parents, or leaders of young children place emphasis on winning, praising the best players and ignoring the others, it makes the others feel even more like "losers."

Recently, physical education has been following a trend to deemphasize competitive sports and to stress instead activities that will help children develop their individual bodies and skills. This is a good thing, because once you have confidence in and control over your body, you can play any game or benefit from any other type of exercise you try.

But if you don't like the idea of sports because you were never a winner, there are still games you can learn; and games, when you enjoy them, don't seem like "exercise"; they just seem like fun. You and a friend could learn tennis (or squash, handball, or golf) together, or you could ask a friend who can play to teach you. You don't have to be the world singles champ; just learn to get the ball over the net and hit it back. These are games that you can play or practice almost anywhere, alone or in a group, and if you keep at them your sports career won't be cut off at the end of high school or college—you'll have a skill and a source of pleasant exercise that will last a lifetime.

There are lots of others. How about bowling? You don't need special equipment unless you want it—just an alley with shoes and balls to rent and a friend who'll give you pointers. Or drag your family away from the television set sometimes for a pickup game of softball or basketball in the park or backyard. Nobody's going to be any good, but who cares? It's fun, and you'll probably have the whole neighborhood or playground wanting to join in, especially if it looks as though nobody's too hung up on winning.

If you can forget about any bad past experience with sports and give games like these (what about archery, skating, skiing, riding?) a try, you may surprise yourself at how well you do when you're not under pressure to be perfect. Even if you don't keep score, you'll be a winner because you'll be getting good, fun exercise.

SINGLES EVENTS

Okay, so maybe you're the kind of person who doesn't like games in any form, no matter how casual. There are still many pleasant ways to get exercise.

Gymnastics can be an immensely satisfying type of vigorous exercise for both boys and girls. It develops muscle tone and demands some endurance, and it helps create graceful coordination. It requires careful training, though, because if you bend or fall the wrong way you can badly dislocate yourself. If the grace and agility of gymnasts intrigues you, see if you can find a class near you to get the basics. Because when you learn how to do it right, you feel as though you're flying—and you often are.

If you are not interested in gymnastics but would like to develop grace and well-shaped muscles, try *modern dancing*. Even the least athletic and most cautious people can enjoy dancing, and you can probably find a class nearby made up of amateurs just like you.

❧ Swimming is nature's most nearly perfect exercise—that is, if you really swim and don't just paddle about in a pool for a while—because it uses all your muscles and expands your heart and lung power without leaving you aching and sweating. The problem with it is that pools are often hard to find close by and year-round; but if a low-cost swimming place is convenient to you, use it often. Swimming is something you can do alone without feeling conspicuous, and you can swim with friends, too. Not only is swimming excellent exercise, it's one that puts you in good touch with your body—you really become aware of the coordination of your muscles, bones, heart, and lungs when you're pushing yourself through the water.

❧ Running and jogging gained great popularity in the mid-1970s, partly because of publicity about heart and lung health, but partly because they could be done in city, suburb, or country and without any skill, training, or fancy equipment. You just need to warm up first, by stretching and walking, and walk yourself "cool" afterwards. You need only one piece of equipment: good shoes. You need the grip and flexibility of running shoes; especially if you have to run on concrete or asphalt rather than grass or dirt, to protect your feet and legs from injuries caused by the shock of slamming your bones against a hard surface; but they don't have to be costly "status" shoes unless that's what you want.

If you feel silly running around the neighborhood by yourself (though lots of people do it) talk a friend into running with you. To a nonjogger, running may sound boring and exhausting. But runners talk glowingly of the sheer joy of feeling their bodies work to capacity, of seeing the world from a different perspective, of meeting new people on their runs. Also, it's the easiest way to get a thorough workout if you do it often enough (at least every other day) and long enough (at least half an hour). So it's worth a try.

Tumbling, dancing, swimming, and running can all be noncompetitive sports. You can do them on your own, if you want, with no winners or losers. But once you get into them, you may find that you are competing against yourself, trying to swim one more length, run one more lap, or do an absolutely perfect back bend. That kind of effort adds to the strength, coordination, and flexibility that these forms of exercise provide, and it also gives you the good feeling of being able to say, if only to yourself, "I did it!" These activities have the added advantage of being lifetime sports (yes, even gymnastics, if you keep at it): with a minimum of equipment you can enjoy them anywhere and any time for the rest of your life.

MAKING EXERCISE A WAY OF LIFE

But maybe you don't have the time or interest to go out for any sports, even the noncompetitive kind. You can still put exercise in your daily life, perhaps in ways you hadn't thought of.

❧ Dance. If you're a person who likes to dance, you're getting good exercise without realizing it when you spend an evening doing some of the more energetic steps. But what if you're not a dancer? Do you avoid school dances or hang around the sidelines if you go? How come? Do you feel dumb dancing, or think you "can't"? Well, all dances are pretty dumb, when you come right down to it, and all of them are pretty easy to learn. Get a friend, brother, or sister to teach you some basic steps and movements, or get a book or do-it-yourself record. Turn on the music, stand in front of a long mirror, and practice.

Pretty soon you'll get the feel of moving your body to the rhythms (and you'll be getting exercise at the same time!). Maybe you aren't perfect, but who cares? If you watch at the next dance you go to (and watching is a good way to learn, too), you'll find that few people are perfect. People admire the really good dancers, but they also enjoy watching and being with somebody who is having a good time without worrying about being perfect. So practice a little and let yourself go—you'll end up with a lot more benefits than getting exercise.

🐾 Walk. Do you demand a ride to the movies, even when they're only a five-minute walk away? Do you pay for a bus ride when you're only going two stops, or take an elevator instead of climbing a couple of flights of stairs? Then you can easily build exercise into your daily routine, and save fuel and money besides: just walk.

Walking works out the muscles, joints, and lungs, and it's good for the soul, too: walking from school can make a rotten day look a lot better by the time you get home. We've become slaves to cars, elevators, and the like, and learning that you can be independent of them can give you a good feeling.

You'll get even more from walking if you stand right when you do it. Good posture helps your body move more efficiently and look better, too. Just standing can be good exercise if you do it right. Holding your stomach flat and the rest of your body in line exercises all the muscles involved.

❧ Posture. Good posture helps any body look better and move more gracefully. Holding yourself well as you walk, sit, or stand also exercises the muscles that are controlling that posture. When you are standing properly, the imaginary line that connects your ear, shoulder, hip, knee, and ankle is straight and perpendicular to the floor: hips and shoulders are *not* thrust back, chin is *not* pointing upward.

Here's how to find your good posture. Grab a few strands of hair at the crown of your head. Pull, and let the rest of your body follow the direction of that pull. Can you feel your body straightening out? Your chin going level? Your ribs lifting off your hipbones? Good. Remember that feeling and try to hold on to it—you'll probably have to exert some effort at first to hold your belly in, keep your shoulders level, or prevent your knees from bending too far forward or backward. But with some practice, you'll develop the muscular control to do that naturally. Stand with the back of your heels and the back of your head flat against a wall. Now press the rest of your body—calves, thighs, spine, shoulders, and neck—against the wall. Take a moment to get the sense of how that feels. Then walk away from the wall, trying to maintain that position. At first you will seem stiff, as though all your torso were in a cast. But if you practice, you'll be able to have that "against the wall" feeling when you are moving normally, and you'll know you're in good shape and alignment.

❧ Work. If you want or need a part-time job, look

for one that makes you move (they're usually the easiest kind for young people to find, anyway). Deliver papers or groceries, wash cars, mow lawns, baby-sit daytimes for young kids, wait tables, clean houses, be a camp counselor—all of those jobs have exercise built into them, and you have the added bonus of being paid while you work out.

Your community probably needs volunteer workers, too. In a hospital, a day-care center, library stacks, or a playground you'll find that you're doing good for yourself and your body as well as for the people you're helping.

❧ Play. How long has it been since you really played? Well, maybe you've outgrown hide-and-seek and red rover; but playing is still fun. The next time you and your friends have "nothing to do" because there's nothing on TV or at the movies, how about biking, or hiking, or rowing, or canoeing? Or sledding, skating, or playing miniature golf or Frisbee? Too many of us have gotten into the habit of watching other people play, and we forget how much fun—and how good for us—it can be to play ourselves.

WORK OUT YOUR OWN WORKOUT

Of course, it is also possible to exercise without ever leaving your own room. And if you're interested in developing or trimming down a specific part of your body, but haven't the time, funds, or interest to join a class or learn a sport, that's probably the best place to do it.

You don't need any equipment—just yourself and an

exercise routine. (See some of the books on page 166 for ideas and instructions.)

If you want a more elaborate setup, get a jump rope (nothing fancy, just a rope heavy enough to swing and long enough to go around your height); some unopened food cans or books of different sizes to serve as weights; a nonslip mat or thick rug; a radio or record player (music makes exercising easier); enough space to swing your arms and legs; your underwear or birthday suit. A pressure pole that you can fit tightly into a doorway is useful for chin-ups or gymnastics—just be sure it's tight, and put cushions on the floor beneath it.

This kind of exercising isn't for everyone. It takes willpower to do it regularly, and it can be boring. But it has the advantages of being private, of accomplishing your specific goals, of costing little or nothing, and of doing something that you can do anywhere and forever.

THE RULES ARE SIMPLE

Whatever kind of fitness program, exercise routine, or game appeals to you, there are a few guidelines to follow.

❧ Enjoy it. If at-home calisthenics, tennis, or whatever is a bore, find something else.

❧ Take it easy. You need to build up gradually toward a goal. Trying to jog five miles the first day would make most people give up that same day; but if they start slow and short, they find that soon those five miles are no trouble at all.

❧ Know what you're doing. You wouldn't dive

into the open ocean if you didn't know how to swim, and you would be foolish to challenge a black-belt karate expert before you had any training. Follow instructions, whether from a teacher or a book.

❧ Warm up and cool off. You need to loosen your joints and warm your muscles before making heavy demands on them, and you need to let your body down gently after you've exercised it. If you're going to jog, walk beforehand and walk afterwards. If you're doing calisthenics, stretch first and hang loose after. A warm shower or bath after strenuous exercise can help you avoid aching muscles.

Some exercise experts say that if your muscles ache after you exercise, you're doing it wrong: that the buildup should be so gradual that you can't feel a thing. Others insist that unless you feel it, you're not working hard enough. So it's up to you—you can take it easy with a painless system or, if you want to feel as though you're getting somewhere, you can push your body harder. Either way, you're getting exercise.

❧ Make it a habit. The more regular exercise is, the more benefit you get from it and the more easily your body adapts to it. You don't have to run or work out every day, but you should establish some regular pattern. Once you get into the exercise habit, you'll find that your body feels uncomfortable when it doesn't get a workout. You won't have to make yourself stretch your legs—you'll want to.

❧ Choose your time. There's a lot of argument about the right time of day to exercise. Some enthusiasts say that morning is the only time, because exercise gets your body going and later in the day you're usually too tired. On the other hand, just getting yourself dressed and out of the house may be all you can manage in the morning. Exercise at night can help you work out a lot of the day's tensions and leave you relaxed and ready for sleep; but if you do vigorous exercises and then hop into bed, you may wake up aching. So again, it's up to you, depending on your own schedule and the kind of program you're following.

❧ Listen to your body. Don't force your body to do something it seems to fight. If you're tired or have a cold or the cramps, take a walk instead of a run, hit a few balls off the backboard instead of playing a tennis game, or do a few stretches instead of a whole series of push-ups. Your body will let you know how much it is able to do—and getting in touch with your body is one of the main benefits of any kind of exercise.

❧ Get it all together. Some forms of exercise have a kind of "mystical" aspect. Most of these are derived from Oriental cultures. Karate, judo, and other martial arts, for instance, we tend to think of as styles of fighting; but they are actually forms of meditation and mental concentration combined with physical activity.

The basic idea behind these forms of exercise is to concentrate one's attention and mental energy fully upon the body part being exercised or the act being performed. In this way, the mind and the body blend.

But you don't need Oriental mysticism to attain this state. When you are doing any kind of exercise, put your whole self into what you are doing. Try doing calisthenics with your eyes closed, shutting out every thing around you. Don't think about your math homework or your love life, but about what your body is doing. Try to feel every move. If you run, concentrate on breathing. Let everything become physical, and somehow magically your mind and spirit will open up. It's the kind of thing that is hard to describe and that you don't believe unless you try it. But bringing your body, mind, and spirit into harmony is one of the many values of finding time for some kind of physical activity.

WHY BOTHER?

If you think that an exercise program, no matter how informal, private, or fun doesn't seem worth the effort, give it another thought.

A physically fit body is one that can get through its daily routine without getting tired, and it also tends to be able to resist stresses of all kinds better than one that is out of shape.

Good exercise will improve your shape by developing your muscles.

It will increase your flexibility and coordination, so that you can make even the simplest motions easily and gracefully. And exercise is a great way to work out your worries and tensions, to get in touch with yourself, and to get all of yourself—body, mind, spirit, and mood—together. That's a good feeling, and it's worth trying to see how good you can feel.

18

TAkE CARE of yourself

When you are feeling good, you are feeling healthy. You are feeling strong enough to meet the demands of your everyday life. You are feeling good about yourself: you like the way you look; you know that there are some things, whether math or cooking or talking, that you do well; you know that you can control your emotions by expressing them in constructive ways.

You can feel good in all these ways by following some new versions of the old familiar rules for health.

❧ "Eat right." Food affects your mind and your moods as much as your physical development. Find out what and how much food your body needs and why, *and* find enjoyable ways to get that nourishment. Nutrition that is good for you needn't be boring.

❧ "Get enough rest." You may get tired of hearing this, but it's still true that a body that is growing and changing as much as yours needs a lot of time off. Fatigue from lack of sleep makes you feel rotten *and* can make your worries and tensions seem a lot worse than they are. But getting enough rest means more than turning out the light when your mother tells you to. Pay attention to your body's needs and your mind's activities; remember that sleeplessness can be caused by tension and that you may need to find and follow your own particular sleeping pattern.

❧ "See your doctor regularly." You need more than checkups; you need a doctor who will listen to you and answer your questions—and you need to be honest with the doctor. Don't be afraid to ask for help from professionals other than your doctor. Nobody can handle every problem alone, and a counselor, "hot line," therapist, or other expert in the social and emotional problems of teen-agers can smooth out a lot of rough spots.

❧ "Don't worry." Everybody worries; the trick is, to get your worries out into the open. If you are concerned about your health or your development, ask the doctor. If you have trouble at school, or at home, or with your friends, talk to someone about it. And remember, no matter how tough it seems to get along with your parents, they are basically on your side—or they want to be once they know what side you're on. The major project of adolescence is to grow away from home and parents, but if you can keep the communication lines open, your parents can help you to do that. Talking may sometimes seem hard, but not talking makes any worry worse.

It may also be worth your while to practice a little

patience. Patience, as you may have heard, is a virtue. Like most virtues, however, it is difficult to attain, especially for someone who can't wait to grow up, who can't wait to look as grown up as his or her friends or to have them be as grown up as he or she is. It may seem that the time will never pass, that you will always look like a little child or be treated as one. But think about it: your change from a child to an adult takes only about five years, and that's a lot less time than you've already been alive. Soon your life—your body, your friends, your social life—will have evened out. That thought might not give you patience, but it could make the waiting seem less painful.

❧ "Live clean." In the old days, when your parents or grandparents were growing up, life was simpler for people your age: drinking, smoking, and sex were absolutely forbidden and therefore almost an impossibility; most illegal drugs weren't even in the picture. Now they are all a lot more available and in some circles acceptable, and that means that you have to make some hard choices. It is important that you *do* choose, that you make a decision based on facts rather than fall blindly into some trap just because "everybody does it." A trap is still a trap even when "everybody" is in it. And you aren't everybody—you are you.

❧ "Get plenty of exercise." Your body will feel better if it is physically fit. But the wrong kind of exercise can be bad for you and your body in many ways. The right kind is something that you enjoy and that helps you to feel comfortable inside your skin. Again, it is a matter of choosing what is right for *you*.

To these should be added a seventh rule for health,

perhaps the most important one: *"Know thyself."* You
need to have knowledge about your personal strengths
and weaknesses so that you can make the most of yourself. You need to understand your moods and feelings
so that you can control and direct them rather than
have them overwhelm you.

The better you understand yourself, the better able
you are to take care of yourself. And it is a good feeling
to be able to take care of yourself.

tHE iNSidE STORY

Here's a quick rundown of your body's parts and how
they work, separately and together. (For more thorough
information, see some of the books listed on page 159.)
The physical "you" consists of billions of tiny *cells*. The
cells are grouped together by type into *tissues*. Tissues
are combined to form *organs*. Several organs working in
conjunction form a *system*. Nine systems operate in the
body.

The *skeletal system* consists of 206 bones connected
by stretchy tissue called ligaments and by cartilage (the
stuff you call gristle when you find it in meat). The
skeleton gives your body its basic shape and provides
protection for the internal organs as well as being a rack
for them to attach to. Also, the marrow, or stuffing, of
many bones is the site for the production of blood cells.

The *muscular system* is what moves those bones and
organs. You have two types of muscles. Striated
("striped") muscles operate the skeleton and, except
for the heart muscles, are under your conscious control.
Smooth muscles make the organs function, and you cannot consciously affect their operation. Tendons—tough,

cordlike connective tissues—attach striated muscles to most bones, and they usually operate in pairs: one to pull a bone in one direction and another to pull it the other way. (Muscles can only pull bones; they cannot push them.) The state of your muscular development also has a lot to do with your shape, since striated muscles bulge under the skin and round off the skeleton.

The *nervous system* makes it possible for those muscles, bones, and organs to operate. About ten billion neurons, or nerve cells, (half of them in the brain) of different types form a network that transmits chemically stimulated electrical signals to and from every part of the body. Sensory nerves send information to specialized portions of the brain (or, in some cases, the main nerve in the spine), which responds by sending action "orders" along motor nerves to the body part involved. This activity is constant and rapid. One segment of the nervous system is automatic; it contains only motor cells and is the means by which the brain keeps the involuntary muscles functioning without your conscious control. But because this segment has links with the portions of the brain that also control emotions, the way you feel can affect the way these nerves act. Anger or fear, for instance, can make the heart beat faster or the digestive system speed up.

The *digestive system*—the esophagus, stomach, intestines, and all the glands that supply those organs with digestive chemicals—processes food into a form that the body's individual cells can use to fuel their operations and maintain themselves. It also provides for the disposal of those parts of your food that the body cannot use.

To convert food into energy, the cells require oxygen, and the supplying of oxygen is the function of the *respiratory system*. When you inhale, air, which is a mixture of gases including oxygen, goes through your mouth and nose into your windpipe, or trachea, and to your lungs. There, the oxygen is filtered from the air and absorbed into the bloodstream. The lungs also take carbon dioxide, the "exhaust" from the cells' functions, out of the blood and force it from the body when you exhale.

The bloodstream flows through the *circulatory system*. Forced through arteries by the pumping action of the heart, blood carries oxygen, nutrients, disease-fighting cells, and other substances to smaller tubes called capillaries where these supplies are exchanged for the cells' waste products. The blood then returns to the heart through the veins and is recycled.

The *lymphatic system* acts as a middleman between the organ tissues in some parts of the body and the circulatory system by exchanging nutrients for waste products. Lymph, the watery fluid that flows through the lymph vessels, is filtered through clumps of cells called nodes, where harmful substances, including bacteria ("germs") are filtered out before the fluid returns to the bloodstream. When some part of the body is diseased, these nodes may become swollen with bacteria, which is why so-called swollen glands are often a symptom of illness.

But lymph nodes are not actually glands. A gland is part of a two-part system of organs that manufactures particular types of fluids. Sweat, saliva, and tears are produced in specific glands of the *exocrine system* and transmitted to the body's surface through tubes called ducts. Important as these glands are to you when you are hot, hungry, or weepy, they are not nearly as important as the glands of the "ductless" or *endocrine system*. The pituitary, thyroid, adrenal, and several other endocrine glands produce chemical substances called hormones which are crucial to the regulation of the body's systems. Transported in the bloodstream, hormones from the various endocrine glands determine your rate of growth, your ability to react in an emergency, the amount of water your body retains, your appetite, the overall efficiency of your bodily processes, your emotional state, and a number of other "minor details" without which you would be a sorry case indeed.

Gonads are endocrine glands that are central to that last-but-not-least system, the *reproductive system*. Male gonads are called testes; female gonads are ovaries. These count as glands because they produce the hormones which regulate the development of secondary sex characteristics that determine how "masculine" or "feminine" a person seems. But gonads are part of the reproductive system because, in a sexually mature body, they also produce the egg or sperm cells necessary for people to reproduce their own kind. The rest of the reproductive system consists of the tubes through which these cells pass, glands to secrete fluids necessary for the process, and, in the female, the uterus. It is in the uterus that a united sperm-and-egg cell, following the pattern set by the genes within the sperm and the egg, begins to divide, add onto itself and differentiate into various types of cells that develop into all the separate tissues, organs and systems that together make a human being.

fuRTHER REAdiNG

... About Your Body and General Health

READ:

Asimov, Isaac. *The Human Body*. Boston: Houghton Mifflin Co., 1963.

A long and detailed explanation for laypeople.

Boston Women's Health Book Collective. *Our Bodies Ourselves* (revised). New York: Simon and Schuster, 1972.

A good roundup on the health problems, needs, and rights of girls and women, including many suggestions for further reading and information sources.

Consumer Reports. *The Medicine Show*. Mt. Vernon, N.Y.: Consumers Union, 1974.

A guide, written for adults, to health problems

and health-care products, giving the facts about such things as acne and colds, debunking the myths, and offering alternatives to highly advertised remedies.

Diagram Group. *Man's Body*. New York: Bantam Books, 1977.

——. *Woman's Body*. New York: Bantam Books, 1978. These "owner's manuals," intended for adults, provide complete guides to the structure, function, needs, and problems of the body. Simply written and clearly illustrated. Facts on nutrition, exercise, and drugs are included. Each book has a section on the opposite sex.

Glimser, Bernard. *All About the Human Body*. New York: Random House, 1958.

Lubowe, Dr. Irwin I. and Barbara Huss. *A Teenager's Guide to Healthy Skin and Hair*. (rev.) New York: Dutton, 1972. About much more than skin and hair, for both boys and girls.

Silverstein, Alvin and Virginia Silverstein. *Sleep and Dreams*. Philadelphia: Lippincott, 1974. A survey of research on sleep and sleep patterns.

Still, Henry. *Of Time, Tides and Inner Clocks*. New York: Pyramid, 1972. Discussion of body rhythms and their influence.

Wilson, Mitchell. *The Human Body*. New York: Golden Press, 1973. An easy-to-read, well-illustrated description of the body's systems and functions.

Zim, Herbert S. *What's Inside of Me?* New York: William Morrow, 1952.

A short, *very* easy-to-read introduction to the body.

. . . All About Aspects of Adolescence

READ:

Collier, James Lincoln. *The Hard Life of the Teenager.* New York: Four Winds, 1972.
Understanding and coping with common problems of adolescence.

Eagan, Andrea Boroff. *Why Am I so Miserable if These Are the Best Years of My Life?* Philadelphia: Lippincott, 1976.
Advice for teen-aged girls.

Gordon, Sol and Roger Conant. *You.* New York: Quadrangle Books, 1975.
An entertaining but factual and sensible presentation of the challenges and conflicts of adolescence.

Mayle, Peter. *What's Happening to Me?* Secaucus, N.J.: Lyle Stuart, 1975.
Wastes too much effort trying to be funny and "with-it," but this is still a clear presentation of the stage of puberty.

. . . About Sex and Related Matters

READ:

Busch, Phyllis. *What About VD?* New York: Four Winds, 1976.
A clearly written, complete book on all forms of V.D.

Chiappa, Joseph A. and Joseph T. Forish. *The V.D. Book*. New York: Holt, Rinehart and Winston, 1976.

Easy-to-read facts from an organization devoted to the study and treatment of V.D.

Dalrymple, Willard, M.D. *Sex Is for Real*. New York: McGraw-Hill, 1969.

A thoughtful, well-written book for teen-agers on all aspects of sex, sexuality, and sexual activity.

Elgin, Kathleen and John F. Osterreicher, M.D. *Twenty-Eight Days*. New York: David McKay, 1973.

A nicely written book about the facts and myths of menstruation.

Gordon, Sol. *Facts About Sex for Today's Youth*. New York: John Day, 1973.

————. *Facts About VD for Today's Youth*. New York: John Day, 1973.

The facts you need to know in clear, readable style.

Guttmacher, Alan F. *Understanding Sex—A Guide for Young People*. New York: Harper and Row, 1970.

Clearly written and sensible.

Horvath, Joan. *What Boys Want to Know About Girls/ What Girls Want to Know About Boys*. New York: Thomas Nelson, 1976.

An interesting presentation of sexual and social information and advice based on interviews with teen-agers.

Hunt, Morton. *Gay: A Young Person's Guide to Homo-*

sexuality. New York: Farrar, Straus & Giroux, 1977.
A calm, factual discussion.

Johnson, Eric W. *Love and Sex in Plain Language* (revised). Philadelphia: Lippincott, 1977.
A basic but thorough book on all aspects of sex.

————. *Sex: Telling It Straight*. Philadelphia: Lippincott, 1970.

Johnson, Eric W. and Corinne Johnson. *Love and Sex and Growing Up*. Philadelphia: Lippincott, 1970.
A very simply written introduction.

Kelly, Gary F. *Learning About Sex*. Woodbury, N.Y.: Barron's, 1976.
A short, complete and up-to-date handbook of the facts.

Loebl, Suzanne. *Conception, Contraception: A New Look*. New York: McGraw-Hill, 1974.
Simply written, thorough survey of the various types of contraception.

Pomeroy, Wardell B. *Boys and Sex*. New York: Dell, 1971.

————. *Girls and Sex*. New York: Dell, 1970.
Classic and still good.

Rosebury, Theodor. *Microbes and Morals*. New York: Viking, 1971.
An interesting account of V.D. and its medical and social effects.

Strain, Frances. *Being Born*. New York: Hawthorne, 1970.
A very simple introduction to the facts of life.

Voelckers, Ellen. *Girls Guide to Menstruation.* New
    York: Richards Rosen, 1975.
    A factual handbook on the subject.
Whelan, Elizabeth M. *Sex and Sensibility.* New York:
    McGraw-Hill, 1974.
    An up-to-date exploration of sex and sexuality
    for young women.
Whelan, Elizabeth M. and E. M. Whelan. *Making Sense
    out of Sex.* New York: McGraw-Hill, 1975.
    An up-to-date exploration of sex and sexuality
    for young men.

CONTACT:

Planned Parenthood Federation of America, Inc.
    810 Seventh Avenue
    New York, N.Y. 10019
    Also has local branches listed in the phone book.
    For information on reproduction and birth con-
    trol.
Sex Information and Education Council of the U.S.
    (SIECUS)
    137 North Franklin Street
    Hempstead, N.Y. 11550
    For referral to sources of information.
U.S. Alliance for the Eradication of VD.
    Philadelphia, Pa.
    Maintains these toll free hotlines for information
    and referral:
        Outside Pennsylvania: 1-800-523-1885
        Pennsylvania, except Philadelphia:
        1-800-462-4966
        Philadelphia area: 567-6969.
U.S. Public Health Service

Maintains or can refer you to V.D. clinics in your area.

... About Your Feelings, Psychology, and Solving Family Problems

READ:

Ewen, Robert B. *Getting It Together*. New York, Franklin Watts, 1976.

An introduction to neuroses and other mental disorders and an explanation of current methods of psychoanalysis.

Hall, Elizabeth. *Why We Do What We Do: A Look at Psychology*. Boston: Houghton Mifflin Co., 1973.

Psychological and emotional motivations for behavior.

Hyde, Margaret O. *Hotline!* New York: McGraw Hill, 1976.

A guide to sources of help for teen-agers in crises.

Hyde, Margaret O. and E. Forsyth. *Know Your Feelings*. New York: McGraw Hill, 1975.

An explanation of emotional states with advice on controlling them. Includes sources for help.

Klagsbrun, Francine. *Psychology—What It Is and What It Does*. New York: Franklin Watts, 1969.

A basic, factual introduction.

———. *Too Young to Die: Youth and Suicide*. Boston: Houghton Mifflin Co., 1976.

A book for and about young people and suicide, with advice on how to find and give help.

LeShan, Eda. *What Makes Me Feel This Way?* New York: Macmillan, 1972.

A simply written book about emotions.

————. *You and Your Feelings.* New York: Macmillan, 1975.
> For teen-agers, the causes of emotional ups and downs.

Marks, Jane. *Help.* New York: Julian Messner, 1976.
> A guide to the various types of counseling and therapy, and a list of some sources of referrals.

Morrison, Carl V., M.D., and Dorothy Morrison. *Can I Help How I Feel?* New York: Atheneum, 1976.
> A guide to understanding and controlling the emotions of adolescence.

Silverstein, Alvin. *Exploring the Brain.* Englewood Cliffs: Prentice Hall, 1973.
> About psychiatry and psychology.

CONTACT:

Family Service Association of America
> 44 East 23rd Street
> New York, N.Y. 10010
> For information on where to find help with family and personal problems in your area.

National Association for Mental Health
> 1800 North Kent Street
> Rosslyn, Va. 22209
> For information on where to find local help in the treatment of mental illness.

... About Nutrition and Weight Control

READ:

American Dietetic Association. *Food Facts Talk Back.*
> Available from the American Dietetic Association, 430 N. Michigan Ave., Chicago, Ill., 60611. An informative, thorough pamphlet.

Berland, Theodore, and the editors of Consumer Guide. *Rating the Diets*. Skokie, Ill.: Publications International, 1974.

A good summary of the various types of reduction diets and the causes and sensible cures for overweight.

Deutsch, Ronald M. *The Family Guide to Better Food and Better Health*. Englewood Cliffs: Prentice Hall, 1964.

A thorough, well-written summary of nutrition and weight control.

Gilbert, Sara. *Fat Free*. New York: Macmillan, 1975.

The author's book for teen-agers on dieting and weight control—how to get rid of fat or stop worrying about it.

————. *You Are What You Eat*. New York: Macmillan, 1977.

The author's book on nutrition and the food business.

Goodhart, R. S. *The Teenager's Guide to Diet and Health*. Englewood Cliffs: Prentice Hall, 1964.

A basic introduction to nutrition.

Jacobson, Michael F. *Nutrition Scoreboard*. New York: Avon Books, 1975.

Information on the quality of the modern diet, and suggestions for getting the most from foods available.

West, Ruth. *The Teenage Diet Book*. New York: Julian Messner, 1969.

A sensible guide to losing weight, including many recipes for low-caloried versions of popular foods.

U.S. Department of Agriculture. *Nutrition: Food at Work for You.*

————. *Food and Your Weight.*

U.S. Department of Health, Education and Welfare. *Facts About Nutrition.*

> The above three booklets are available from the Superintendent of Documents, U.S. Government Printing Office, Washington, DC, 20402.

. . . About Drugs, Alcohol, and Cigarettes

READ:

Creative Learning Group. *All About Drugs.* Cambridge, Mass.: Media Engineering Corporation. 1970.

> A set of pamphlets organized so that you can teach yourself about the properties and effects of all types of drugs.

Engelbardt, Stanley L. *Kids and Alcohol, the Deadliest Drug.* New York: Lothrop, 1975.

> Detailed description of the effects of alcohol.

Gorodetzky, Charles W. and Samuel T. Christian. *What You Should Know About Drugs.* New York: Harcourt, Brace, Jovanovich, 1970.

> A sensible, factual presentation.

Greenberg, Harvey R., M.D. *What You Should Know About Drugs and Drug Abuse.* New York: Four Winds, 1970.

> A calm and readable book for young people.

Houser, Norman W. and J. B. Richmond. *Drugs: Facts on Their Use and Abuse.* New York: Lothrop, 1969.

> Simply written, matter-of-fact information.

Hyde, Margaret O., Editor. *Mind Drugs.* New York: McGraw-Hill, 1974.
> Experts describe the effects and dangers of each type of drug.

Langone, John. *Bombed, Buzzed, Smashed, or Sober.* Boston: Little, Brown, 1976.
> The pros and cons of alcohol use.

Madison, Arnold. *Drugs and You.* New York: Julian Messner, 1971.
> A simply written book for young readers.

Public Affairs Committee. *Alcoholics and Alcoholism.* (no. 426).

———. *Drug Abuse: What Can Be Done?* (no. 390A).

———. *Cigarettes.* (no. 439A).

———. *What About Marijuana?* (no. 436).
> The above pamphlets are short, factual, and easy to read. Available from Public Affairs Pamphlets, 381 Park Ave. South, New York, N.Y. 10016.

Silverstein, Alvin and V. B. Silverstein. *Alcoholism.* Philadelphia: Lippincott, 1975.
> The causes and effects of alcoholism. Includes a chapter on living with an alcoholic parent.

U.S. Department of Health, Education, and Welfare. *Drinking Etiquette.*
> Good advice on how to—and how not to—drink politely.

———. *The Drinking Question.*
> About (rather than for or against) drinking, written for teen-agers.

> The above two booklets are available from the Superintendent of Documents, U.S. Government Printing Office, Washington, D.C., 20402.

CONTACT:

Alcoholics Anonymous, Alanon, Alateen.
>Check your phone book for local branches of these associations for alcoholics and their families.

American Association of Health, Physical Education and Recreation,
>1201 Sixteenth Street, N.W.
>Washington, D.C. 20036
>This organization provides information on smoking, drinking, and drug abuse.

American Cancer Society, Inc.
>219 East 42nd Street
>New York, N.Y., 10017
>(or see phone book for local chapter)
>For information on smoking and how to quit.

National Clearinghouse for Alcohol Information
>Box 2345
>Rockville, Md. 20852

National Clearinghouse for Drug Abuse Information
>5600 Fishers Lane
>Rockville, Md. 20857

National Council on Alcoholism, Inc.
>733 Third Avenue
>New York, N.Y. 10017

. . . About Exercise

READ:

American Medical Association. *Basic Bodywork.* Available from American Medical Association, Order Department OP-428, 535 N. Dearborn Street, Chicago, Ill. 60610.

A good pamphlet outlining basic but thorough exercises for both sexes and summarizing requirements for fitness and general health.

Bendick, Jeanne and Marcia Levin. *Pushups and Pinups*. New York: McGraw-Hill, 1963.

Diet, exercise, and grooming for boys and girls. Easy reading.

Cooper, Dr. J. Kenneth. *The New Aerobics*. New York: Bantam Books, 1970.

This and the earlier *Aerobics* are good guides to the safe way of getting the most out of vigorous exercise.

Delza, Sophia. *Body and Mind in Harmony*. New York: David McKay, 1961.

A good introduction to the Oriental art of T'ai Chi.

Frankel, Lillian and Godfrey. *Muscle-building Games*. New York: Gramercy Press, 1964.

Simple exercises, mainly for boys.

Getchel, Bud. *Physical Fitness—A Way of Life*. New York: John Wiley, 1976.

A simply written discussion of the benefits and requirements of overall physical fitness, including instructions for vigorous exercises and warm-ups.

Giles, Frank. *Toughen Up*. New York: G. P. Putnam's Sons, 1963.

Step-by-step fitness and bodybuilding guide for boys, including weightlifting.

Hoffman, Bob. *Weight Training for Athletes*. New York: Ronald Press, 1961.

Good instruction in weightlifting techniques for non-athletes as well.

Jacobs, Helen Hull. *Better Physical Fitness for Girls.* New York: Dodd, Mead, 1964.
Exercise routines and general health advice.

Kiss, Michaeline. *Yoga for Young People.* Indianapolis: Bobbs-Merrill, 1971.
A clear introduction to yoga as exercise.

Leonard, George. *The Ultimate Athlete.* New York: Viking, 1975.
A well-written book about the new style of physical education and the need for lifetime sports. Includes suggestions for a variety of physical activities that are both fun and worthwhile.

Lettvin, Maggie. *The Beautiful Machine.* New York: Alfred A. Knopf, 1972. In paperback, New York: Ballantine, 1975.
The best available guide to indoor exercises, providing detailed instructions for programs designed to shape up, strengthen, increase flexibility, and treat and prevent physical problems, for both sexes. The "hardcover" consists of individual instruction cards with a separate index pamphlet; the soft-cover offers the same exercises, but without the convenience of the cards, which allow you to easily organize your own "system."

Lewis, Nancy and Richard Lewis. *Keeping in Shape.* New York: Franklin Watts, 1976.
An easy-to-read guide to exercise and fitness.

Morehouse, Laurence E. and Leonard Gross. *Total Fit-*

ness in 30 Minutes a Week. New York: Pocket Books, 1976.

The "30 minutes a week" of the title is misleading, but the book does offer a complete guide to total fitness, based mainly on the "aerobics" system, but including a number of other suggestions for exercise.

President's Council on Physical Fitness and Sports. *Fit For Life*.

A good short guide to nutrition and exercise, especially jogging.

————. *Vigor*.

————. *Vim*.

Booklets outlining simple but thorough exercise plans: *Vigor* is "for boys"; *Vim* is "for girls."

————. *Youth Physical Fitness*.

This booklet is written for school physical education programs, but it provides detailed instructions on exercises that will help young readers of both sexes develop strength, grace, and stamina.

These four publications are available from The President's Council on Physical Fitness and Sports, Washington, D.C., 20201 or from the U.S. Government Printing Office, Washington, D.C., 20402.

Prudden, Bonnie. *Teenage Fitness*. New York: Harper & Row, 1965.

A thorough, sensible program from a competent expert.

Schneider, Tom. *Everybody's a Winner*. Boston: Little, Brown, 1976.

> Suggestions for fun, noncompetitive exercise and games.

Schultheis, Ingrid. *Slimming with Weights*. San Francisco: San Francisco Book Co., 1977.

> "Weightlifting" for girls, based on a YMCA program.

Simon, Ruth Bluestone. *Relax and Stretch*. New York: Collier Books, 1975.

> A simple, complete program combining yoga and nonvigorous "western" exercises.

Turner, Alice K. *Yoga for Beginners*. New York: Franklin Watts, 1973.

> A good, easy-to-read introduction to the theory and practice of yoga.

YMCA. *The Official YMCA Physical Fitness Handbook*. New York: Popular Library, 1977.

> A thorough program designed for strength, stamina and flexibility; aimed at both sexes.

CONTACT:

American Association for Health, Physical Education and Recreation.

> 1201 Sixteenth Street, N.W.
> Washington, D.C. 20036

President's Council on Physical Fitness and Sports.

> Washington, D.C. 20201

YMCA

YWCA

> Check your phone book for the address and number of your local chapter.

index